WHAT PEOPLE ARE SAYING ABOUT
40 DAYS TO PERSONAL REVOLUTION

"The forty days program peels away the obstacles that stand between you and your greater growth."

—Alice R.

"Register for this program when you're feeling lost and unmotivated. It'll give you a renewed sense of self and restart the flames you've lost."

—Arby C.

"Not sure I can put it all into words other than the result is profound. It is life-changing if you apply the principles and commit to the program."

—Brandy B.

"It was life-changing for me."

—Bruce P.

"*40 Days to Personal Revolution* helped me to be OK with showing up and being OK with what is. I'm a very competitive person, more so with myself. So a lot of times in programs it's ready set go, push push push! This program was ready set be, breathe, and see!"

—Carla J.

"A wonderful way to get in the groove of eating in a more balanced way, get moving in new ways with themed yoga practices and investigate my belief systems and updating them through the inquiry questions provided, and a deep letting go and awakening through meditation."

—Cindy L.

"It allowed me to step away and examine areas of my life that I had some blind spots that were holding me back. With awareness, I can now address those areas and move forward in expansion. Great program that shines new light on areas you had no clue that were holding you back from your Greatness."

—Christen S.

"The forty days program gave me renewed skills to deal with difficulties in my life. I feel stronger emotionally and physically."

—Christine W.

"This was and is a (as I quote *The Shawshank Redemption*) 'Either get busy living or get busy dying' experience."

—Colette R.

"I found this program to be such a great guide to truly tapping into the whole picture. Guiding me through each step of personal growth and considering all areas of my life that could be examined, fine-tuned, and guided to find success for growth while applying the steps of this program. It is truly amazing to experience this program's results when you follow the steps as a guide . . . everything falls into place. Even if you don't do it perfectly; there is an awareness that unfolds that gives you a sense of accomplishment that is guilt free!!!"

—Doreen R.

"*40 Days to Personal Revolution* allowed me to connect to and be supported as I embarked on a program of yoga, meditation, reflection, and nutrition. I loved feeling part of something that brought out a bigger and better version of me."

—Glen H.

"*40 Days to Personal Revolution* challenged and inspired me to regain my power, purpose, and true self. I committed to the work and the process worked on me. I finish my forty days with the gift of knowing that this is not an end but a continuing journey of exploration and revelation. I don't have to arrive anywhere. Thank you."

—Helwen C.

"This program can be life-changing and I highly recommend it!"

—Jodi B.

40 Days

to Personal

Revolution

A Breakthrough Program to Radically Change Your Body and

Awaken the Sacred Within Your Soul

Baron Baptiste

Photographs by Richard Corman

ATRIA PAPERBACK

New York   London   Toronto   Sydeny   New Delhi

ATRIA
PAPERBACK

An Imprint of Simon & Schuster, Inc.
1230 Avenue of the Americas
New York, NY 10020

This Atria Paperback edition June 2022

ATRIA PAPERBACK and colophon are trademarks of Simon & Schuster, Inc.

For information about special discounts for bulk purchases, please contact Simon & Schuster
Special Sales at 1-866-506-1949 or business@simonandschuster.com.

The Simon & Schuster Speakers Bureau can bring authors to your live event.
For more information or to book an event, contact the Simon & Schuster Speakers Bureau
at 1-866-248-3049 or visit our website at www.simonspeakers.com.

Interior design by Ruth Lee-Mui

Manufactured in the United States of America

1   3   5   7   9   10   8   6   4   2

Library of Congress Cataloging-in-Publication Data is available.

ISBN 978-1-6680-0211-7
ISBN 978-0-7432-5390-1 (ebook)

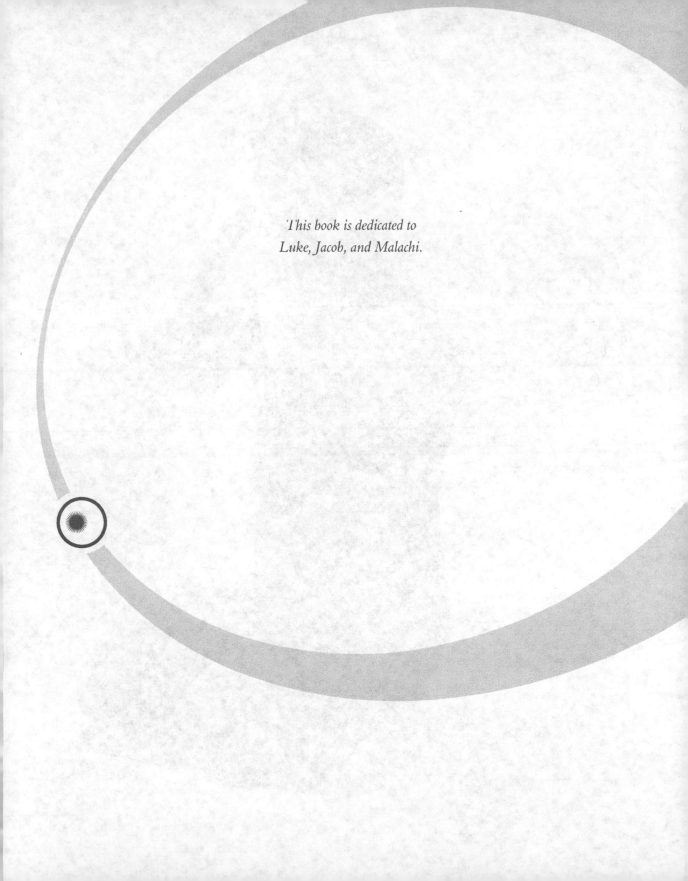

This book is dedicated to
Luke, Jacob, and Malachi.

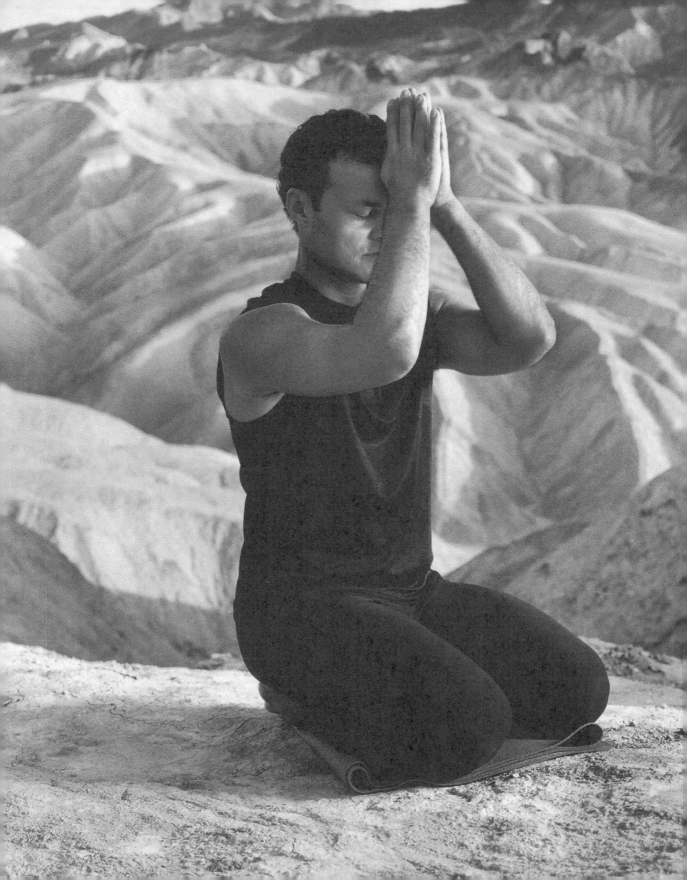

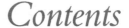

Contents

Acknowledgments

Thank you to my literary agent, Ling Lucas. Thank you to Magana Baptiste, Jesse Peterson, Robert Traynor, and Coeli Marsh. I thank Debra Goldstein, my brilliant wordsmith (and good friend). To Ken Rosen for his insights and input into the principles of sound nutrition.

To Caroline Sutton, whose experienced eye and commitment to excellence brought all of the components of this book together.

Once again a heartfelt thanks to Richard Corman, who shot the photographs in this book with skill and an eye for excellence. Also thank you to Richard's assistants, Peter Chin and Jackson Lynch, and to Caroline Bradley. To Nadja Jenkins for sharing her joy-filled yoga practice in the pictures of this book

A huge thank-you to Ken Browning for his ongoing support, guidance, and expertise in making this and many other projects a reality. To Mark Aronchik and David Pudlin: your unending insight and guidance has been a blessing. To Jim Meade for his expertise and experienced opinion.

To my entire teaching team at the Baptiste Power Yoga Institutes and our affiliate studios around the world who diligently carry forth this powerful work and maintain the integrity of the vision. Your contribution is self evident. I salute you.

Thank you to the whole team of behind-the-scenes folks at Simon & Schuster, who worked day and night to complete this book, especially Christine Lloreda, Laurie Cotumaccio, Debbie Model, Marcia Burch, and Cherlynne Li.

I am very grateful to my loyal and steadfast managers at BPYI offices, who faithfully work day in and day out in order to bring me to Bootcamps and workshops all over the world that are overflowing with enthusiastic students. To Vyda Bielkus, who remains constantly committed to the vision that what we are doing does make a difference and that by helping our community grow to new levels, we grow as people.

And most of all, thanks to every person who has read *Journey into Power,* attended my classes, workshops, and/or followed a video or CD and shared with me and/or others the powerful testimony of the value this work has had in their lives. Their support for this work means more to me than I could possibly put into words.

And most important—I thank God.

ACKNOWLEDGMENTS

New Introduction to

40 DAYS TO PERSONAL REVOLUTION

Life is a journey, but at a certain point in any journey what is needed is a reset. The fact that you are holding this book in your hands means you're being called to take a new path, a new kind of journey from wherever you are in your life right now. Something within you is pulling you toward a new way, a new possibility. A pull toward new ways of living, a pull toward what's possible in your physical and mental well-being and health. It could be something deep within you that's calling you to live from a truer place in your heart or from a deeper space of faith and trust in a spiritual power.

I'm reminded of a woman who shared with me during a *40 Days to Personal Revolution* program that she was doing the program for a second time. I asked, why do it again? She explained that a year and a half ago she was out

for a run with her dog and was hit by a drunk driver. This resulted in multiple broken bones and some brain trauma. As a result of this accident she lost her job and fell into living in a world full of fear and uncertainty about her health and financial future. She turned to food as a way to comfort herself and quickly put on forty-plus pounds that felt unhealthy to her. Nine months after her accident she signed up for 40 Days to Personal Revolution online program that I was leading. It was the disruption she needed. The daily yoga practices along with the cleansing diet provided a renewed sense of physical strength and vitality and put her on track to lose all the weight she had put on. She felt lighter and brighter for the first time in over a year and a half. She said about twenty days into the program she put more attention on practicing the spiritual principles, journaling, and meditations that resulted in a powerful shift in mindset. She said that after completing the program she dived right back into life head-on. She took on rock climbing, skiing, went back to school and got her master's degree. She even signed up for a leadership course with me. She went on to say that *40 Days to Personal Revolution* was the disruption and precise guidance she needed to start living fully again.

We are on a journey from the day we were born, and it won't end until our time on earth is complete. The question for each of us is what kind of journey will it be? We can't change the past, however with the practices in this book, and perhaps some help from a higher power, you do have some say in how the future will go for you. At certain points through our journey in life we get stuck, lose our way, we feel the world is full of resistance. It is at these points on our journey that we need a refresh—a personal revolution. Better than anyone, you know your strengths and weaknesses, your failures and successes, and your heartaches. But the truth is we don't have to be shackled by the past. Instead, as the prophets and teachers of old have promised, there is always a way to begin anew. Consider there is a power within you that wants you to be happy, healthy, and stress-free. This power within you, is the authentic YOU.

The authentic you has a natural commit-ment to change and grow, what the 40 Days to Personal Revolution program does is give structure to fulfill that commitment that's already within your power. This program supports you in disrupting old ways of being and acting and puts your feet on a new path—an empowered path. This is what this book is all about, and this is what I invite you to do. This book has urged the thousands of people who have taken this program before you, to start with just forty days of practice in order to choose a new path—a different path from the one you've been on. This path is one which we will each ultimately choose for ourselves but this program is in-tended to support you in starting anew and supports you in living true. As we choose to take a personal revolution, our journey in life will continue, but now you will be on a path that rings true. Why take it? Why take a new path now? Why not stay on the road we already know? Even if we haven't yet found the inner peace, vitality, power, and free-dom we have been wanting all of our lives, isn't it easier to stay with what we know?

After witnessing thousands of people en-gage in their own personal revolution and with profound results, let me give you two powerful reasons to consider why changing to a new path *now* is worth the risk.

First, the old path will never deliver what it promises. Even if the old path has deliv-ered on promises in the past, over time the old path becomes no longer fulfilling and satisfying, it can become deadening.

For many people, the old path promised fulfillment, joy, and security—but ends up in anxiety, fear, heartache, boredom, and anguish. The old path probably promised freedom too—but ended up enslaving us with stress, resentment, and bitterness.

There are endless examples in life of those who chose the wrong path, thinking it was the right one—and in one way or another it led to disappointment, or worse.

For many of us, the old path promised us everything, but it's promises ended up being hollow and left us feeling empty. A good question to ask ourselves is why stay on the old path we've been on if it no longer is giving us the results we want?

Please don't misunderstand me. I'm not saying our journey always will be easy and trouble free if you simply do the program in this book. Life is just not like that. We can do all of the physical and spiritual practices on this side of heaven and it won't make us exempt from suffering and grief. However, in doing our part, there is the real possibility that amidst all of life's difficulties and challenges we can still experience inner peace, power, and freedom in the face of life's troubles. Not because we're lucky, but because we have practiced.

The second reason for choosing a new path that is of supreme importance: *it leads us home.* Because of this new path, whenever I am traveling, I constantly look forward to the moment when I will return home. Even if I'm full-on busy and preoccupied leading a program, training, or giving a talk, somewhere in the back of my mind one thought is always present; "soon I get to be going home!" Home is a place of security, rest, and where we get to be fully ourselves; home is where we belong. Home is where the heart is.

Although our physical home might represent all of that, what I am pointing to here is something much deeper and more profound than our physical house and home. In fact, I'm not speaking about physical things at all. I'm speaking about the importance of being at home in our own skin, at home in our own hearts—*being at home in ourselves.* There is a natural power and confidence that comes from being at home within ourselves—wherever we may be. Taking the new path means finding your new home in yourself and always wanting to go back.

We each know when it's time for a change, a true change. In the last twenty years thousands of people have taken this *40 Days to Personal Revolution* pathway, I believe that you will have the experience of "coming home" and realize the possibility of *living true* in your body, mind and being.

Let the revolution begin!
Baron Baptiste
December 2021

40 Days
to Personal
Revolution

PART ONE

The Laws of Transformation

The Foundation of Your Revolution

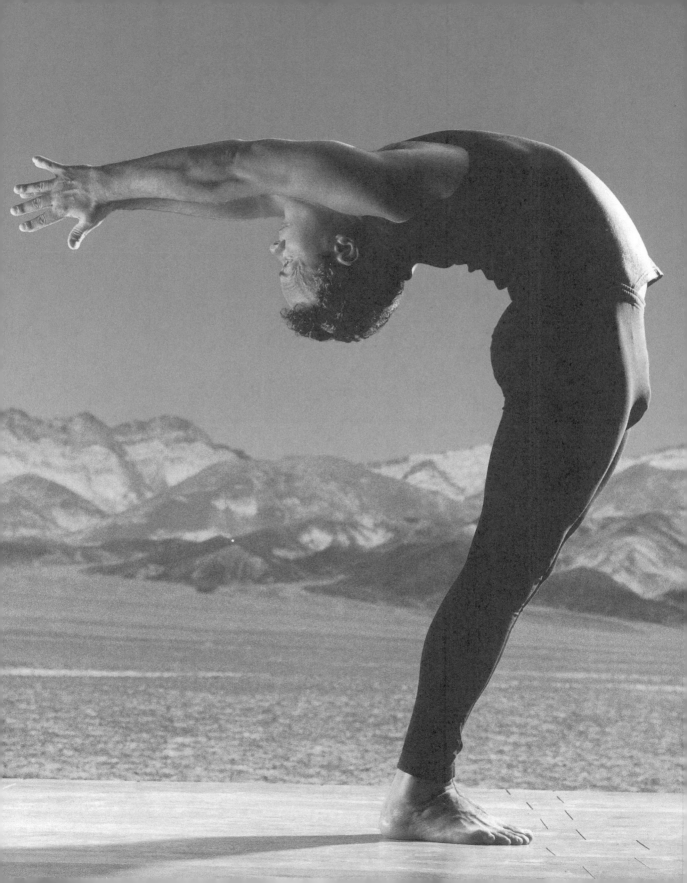

ACCORDING TO GANDHI, HEALTH MUST BE SOUGHT PRIMARILY IN THE REALM OF THE SPIRIT, THROUGH A THOUGHTFUL OBSERVANCE OF THE LAWS OF NATURE. HE

believed that as whole, interconnected beings, we can trace any lack of health we experience to mental and spiritual causes, and that vitality and health can be transformed only when a person's entire attitude toward life is changed. In his wisdom, he knew that what was necessary for true health was to live by the laws of nature in relationship to diet, purposeful exercise, fresh air, positive surroundings, forgiveness, and a pure heart.

Although we are calling the laws here the Laws of Transformation, they could also be called the laws of nature or the laws of life, because these same timeless and universal principles hold true in all these realms. Like physical laws, there are spiritual laws that govern the universe. And like the law of gravity, spiritual laws of transformation exist whether we believe in them or not. Our votes mean nothing. This is why, as you will discover in Law 4, we must hold a space within ourselves for faith.

The laws here are principles by which we can live and grow. They can act as the guiding beacon of light on the high road toward truth and whole-life health. The more closely we cleave to these principles and natural laws, the more effortlessly we will be changed. To the degree that we choose to live by them, our life flows. To the degree that we reject them, we struggle.

When we violate the laws of nature, we are not living up to our potential. It doesn't necessarily mean we are bad, just that we are not entirely in the know. When you have an innate knowledge of these laws within your consciousness, however, it gives you the ability to create a flow of energy and light in your life, which allows you to tap new realms of physical transformation and spiritual evolution. You are no longer swimming upstream, and as a result, you feel more at home in your body and at peace with the pressures of your life.

When we look at anything through the perspective of principles, we immediately shift our perception to the bigger picture. There is a greater purpose and meaning behind what we are doing, and we are led by a higher force rather than just haphazardly taking action. Without principles, we are subject to anarchy and chaos. All the pieces of this program mean nothing if they are not undertaken in the spirit of these laws. There is a saying in the Bible that "a foolish man builds his house on sand." By understanding, internalizing, and living these timeless principles, we are building our house on rock, and from this foundation, we can flow and grow into true success in life.

All of the Laws of Transformation are interconnected. The laws depend on each other, and like the cells of one body, they work together toward a greater meaning. I encourage you to read these all the way through, to establish your philosophical foundation for your forty-day journey, and then to return to them as you proceed through the weeks. Something that may not have made sense to you in the beginning may take on a wholly different meaning as you go through the process. I believe that you intuitively already know these principles, and therefore they will resonate with you and will reinforce what you already knew in your heart. As Socrates said, "True learning is remembering."

The Twelve Laws of Transformation

LAW 1: Seek the Truth

LAW 2: Be Willing to Come Apart

LAW 3: Step out of Your Comfort Zone

LAW 4: Commit to Growth

LAW 5: Shift Your Vision

LAW 6: Drop What You Know

LAW 7: Relax with What Is

LAW 8: Remove the Rocks

LAW 9: Don't Rush the Process

LAW 10: Be True to Yourself

LAW 11: Be Still and Know

LAW 12: Understand That the Whole Is the Goal

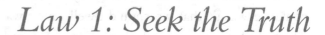

Law 1: Seek the Truth

Then you will know the truth, and the truth will set you free.

—JOHN 8:31–33

A MAN WHO WAS LIKE AN UNCLE TO ME WAS A BRAHMACHARYA (A YOGIC RENUNCIATE). HE HAD BEEN THE RIGHT-HAND MAN TO THE FAMOUS YOGA GURU

Yogananda for about twenty years before he went on to discover a new path. I remember when I was in my late teens I had a conversation with him that was so profound, I immediately went and wrote it down, word for word, so that I could remember it. It began when I asked him how I could get unstuck from the world of competition that seemed to create so much fear and suffering in my life.

He nodded understandingly. "That particular question and a thousand others pertaining to the human predicament can be answered with one word. It's an ancient word found in almost every spiritual tradi-

tion that is now glibly tossed from a hundred thousand pulpits every Sunday of each week. Because of such familiarity, it's been cheapened, and its deeper mystical meaning has been lost."

I said, "Please, tell me—what's the word?"

"Repentance."

"Oh," I said, the sneer on my face making it very clear that the word had associations for me. Quite frankly, whenever I heard that word, aside from its rather distasteful religious connotation, shivers would go up my spine, and I always got the image of a magazine cartoon showing a

5

bearded elder in a white robe and sandals walking the streets of Manhattan with a sign saying Repent! The End of the World Is Near.

He and I talked some more, and I came to understand that what he meant by repentance wasn't that we should dwell on where we lost our way and all the ways we are bad, but rather to have the courage to face the pure, unsweetened truth of ourselves so that we can move on and grow in more honest and authentic ways. It is simply the willingness to see in full truthfulness what we need to face within ourselves and our lives so that we may get into the right alignment. As Jesus taught, it is ultimately always the truth that can set us free.

I have since come to believe that the highest form of repentence is self-acceptance. As the philosopher Carl Rogers said, "The curious paradox is that when I accept myself just as I am, then I can change." You can meditate and do yoga until you are blue in the face, and all you will ever be is blue in the face unless you have the courage to open your heart, face reality, admit your mistakes, and take right action. It hurts a bit, but this is what it means to have a personal revolution.

Not too many years after this conversation, I went through a personal awakening in which I started to feel like I had wasted much of my life on futile things. In the process, I saw how I had hardened my heart, and it pained me. I saw all the ways I had missed the mark. I felt like my heart was cracking open—and I cried as I saw how I'd been wasting my life being prideful, unforgiving, and ungrateful, isolated from myself and the people in my life. I was genuinely sorry about it. I was deeply sad, yet profoundly glad to see these things about myself, because I knew it was an opportunity for a new birth, a new beginning in life.

There is a Turkish proverb that says, "No matter how far you have gone down a wrong road, turn back," and that is exactly what I did. It was painful, but also one of the most beautiful things I have ever experienced. When the truth entered my heart, it was as though a thousand pounds of emotional weight had been lifted. Much karma was burned in this sacred moment. For me, this was an authentic and conscious experience of growth in my life.

That was an experience that opened something deep in me. It was as if there was a powerful energy system that broke through the membrane that was holding me back in life. Have you ever felt like "Here's my power, here's my energy and strength, here are my talents, here is the gift that I was meant to give"—but then there is an invisible membrane that blocks all this from shining through?

In the religious East they say that if you have done a wrong in the past, it has to be undone. And so perhaps this breaking through is needed in order to see the truth, remap your mind, and establish a new direction. The remapping occurs in the silence of our hearts. Alone and absolutely empty, we acknowledge that there is a lack of right direction and that we need to repent so that we may be rebuilt. The ego will feel that in this deep surrender life ends, but truly, it's the point where life begins.

Law 2: Be Willing to Come Apart

One must lose one's life in order to find it.

—ANNE MORROW LINDBERGH

SOMEONE ONCE ASKED JESUS, "WHAT IS HEAVEN?"

"HEAVEN IS LIKE THE MUSTARD SEED," HE REPLIED. THOUGH THE mustard seed is among the tiniest of seeds, he explained, it one day grows into the largest of trees. Like heaven—and like us—its potential is vast.

We are all like this tiny seed. We all have flashes of awareness in which we realize that who we are in all our smallness has essentially to break apart in order for a new self to emerge. It's as though something whispers in our ear, "I can't continue this way." Those moments can panic us into reaching out for another false balm (a drink, a drug, a snack, a pat on the back, a chocolate), or they can light the sparks of revolution and be catalysts for us to break apart so that we may emerge, like a seed becoming a tree, in a wholly new form.

There is a lot of value in being willing to completely come apart. We can give up the illusion that everything is okay and that we can control anything, and begin our true spiritual work. There is so much in life we can't control. When we control, we are playing God. In the Taoist religions they refer to God as an energy. There is a higher power and flow of the universe—they call it the Tao—that holds everything together, gives order, and creates a beautiful orchestration of nature. Flow is not an empty phenomenon or a psychological construct; it has an incredible genius and ingenuity that harmonizes all things into a sophisticated ecosystem of goodness that works. Look at a cell that becomes an embryo that ultimately becomes a baby. Look at how planets revolve around the sun and how the solar system is set up. We don't need to be an Einstein to recognize that there is an intelligence at work. Yet the limited ego mind thinks that this applies to everything except us. We want to control our lives ourselves. Many of us arrogantly think we need to be in charge, even though, as *A Course in Miracles* says of this greater intelligence, "I who hold galaxies together could handle the little circumstances of your life."

For many of us, we need to get to the point where we are finally willing to give up control so that we can experience the healing we so desperately need. Sometimes our body becomes ill because it just can't hold it all together any longer. Falling ill forces us to stop, slow down, and give up our drive so that healing can occur. In order for the body's healing system to take over, we need to trust and lose control, just as we do when we fall asleep at night. It's as though we hand ourselves over to the forces of nature to be restored, recharged, and renewed. That is why control freaks are usually insomniacs; they simply can't let go.

We have a hard time with surrender. To many of us, surrender means "I lose." The truth is that we can afford to relax and surrender because it's not a loss at all. In fact, it's a win. When we control the things that we are not meant to control, we are interfering with our natural success and potential.

The truth is that we are not stable, but the Tao is. Trying to control all the instability and uncertainty of life is crazy-making and exhausting, and it creates disease. No matter what the circumstances happen to be, the way of the universe is for all things to move in the direction of healing, that is, wholeness. The body wants to heal itself, our emotional body is seeking balance, our spirit wants redemption; however, we need to get ourselves out of the way in order for our natural health to shine through. We need to totally lose control, and this scares the heaven out of us.

We are always fighting. We are fighting for the job, we're fighting for the relationship, we're fighting our partner or parents to be a certain way, we're fighting to maintain our fixed agendas. We're fighting to get people to understand us, we're fighting to get our body a certain way, we're fighting to make money, we're fighting to avoid failure, we're fighting for the next success, we're fighting to be what we think we should be. All this fighting hardens us, contracts us, and makes us sick. Fighting has to do with getting. And a *get* state of mind is not a healthy state of mind. When we put out a *get* mentality, we'll be *got*. But when we relax, we receive.

I know that in my own life, whenever I fight and struggle to make anything happen, it backfires. The energy gets blocked, as does the ultimate manifestation of good in that circumstance. When I give up the struggle in any area of my life, I see how things unfold. When things work out on my behalf, I didn't *make* them happen; I *allowed* them to happen.

In our lives, like in our bodies, if we refuse to give up control, life will eventually do it for us. Controlling the flow of life is like setting up a dam: All the flow stops, and it builds up within us as pressure. Finally it breaks and brings us to our knees, and we hit a crisis. Crisis can be a call to spiritual rebirth. We get sick, lose our jobs or someone close to us, or experience a clear and painful moment seeing something about ourselves, and suddenly the ice around our heart breaks. At the crossroads we can shut down and get resentful, or we can break up, break with, and break through to new ground. This point at the crossroads is a spiritual test.

Buddha said that suffering is inevitable as long as we believe that things will last— that they don't fall apart, and we can count on them. From Jesus's point of view, the only time we ever really know the truth of life is when the rug has been pulled out from underneath us. At different points in my life, I've been driven to a place where everything fell apart. All the ways I isolated myself, all the ways I deluded myself, and all the ways I maintained a well-polished image splintered into thousands of tiny pieces. No matter what I tried, I simply could no longer hold it all together, and the dam broke. Painful and humbling as they were, those were the moments in which I found wisdom and strength. I've learned that it is only when we are willing to give up the fragile hold we have on our illusions and come apart that we can begin to see the truth, surrender, and begin anew.

Law 3: Step out of Your Comfort Zone

The easy path leads to the hard life, but the hard path leads to the easy life.

—RILKE

THE QUESTION FOR ANYONE ON A JOURNEY OF TRANSFORMATION IS NOT "WILL I SURVIVE IF I STEP OUT OF MY COMFORT ZONE?" THE REAL QUESTION IS "WILL I

survive my comfort zone?"

The comfort zone may feel cozy and familiar, but it is like sweet poison, silently killing off our childlike spontaneity and our vitality. When we choose our comfort zone over growth we get stuck or worse, because ultimately we are either awakening and growing or numbing out and spiraling downward. Life is never static—we either grow or we die.

A comfort zone is a state of mind, body, and soul that we reach out to when we find ourselves unable to deal properly with the pressures of the world. It is a place we can go to coast in life and not have to face the challenges that arise. The doorway to the zone is anything that affects us emotionally—confusion, anger, fear, or the primal need to escape. But by escaping into a comfort zone, we render ourselves vulnerable to all kinds of sabotaging behavior, addiction, and stagnation.

Stepping out of our comfort zone means dropping the patterns and stories of the past. Our patterns don't have to go on forever; we can leave the past behind us if we are truly willing. If we don't step out of the known—the comfort zone—we bring yesterday's limited thinking into the present, therefore dooming the present to be just like the past. We will keep repeating and doing the same things again and again, getting the same results, and then complain, "Nothing ever changes in my life." We gather evidence to justify all the things that we bring into the present with us. We seek proof of why we *can't* change, and all kinds of reasons why we *won't* let go of our dramas, stresses, resentments, fears, or self-destructive ways of being.

So many of us would rather cling to the familiar than risk the unknown. The past is familiar, something we can hold on to, while the future is completely uncharted and feels groundless. But we must venture forward in order to grow. Jesus taught his students to walk toward their fears with an open heart rather than away from them, to face them head-on so that we can dissolve their hold over us.

Often, stepping out of our comfort zone has more to do with the simplicity of forgiveness and self-honesty than it does with a grandiose breaking out of some box. There is a Zen story about a monk who told his teacher that the breathing meditation that was prescribed for him was boring. "Don't you have any interesting meditations?" he asked his teacher. The master grabbed the student, pushed him into a lake, and held him underwater. The student kicked and struggled for air and tried to get up for a long time. Finally after a minute or two the teacher let him up.

"How was it?" the master said.

"Terrible," said the student. "I couldn't breathe!"

The Zen master replied, "Yes, but your breath became very interesting to you!"

If we live according to the past, we are bound to feel anguish, boredom, and a kind of meaninglessness. The comfort zone has its own kind of consciousness that is aware that you have become redundant, that you are doing the same habitual pattern again and again and will be doing it tomorrow, too. This is a dilemma we all face in life, and the only solution is to let the past die. There is a beautiful story of the life of Jesus in which he comes to a fishing village and sees a fisherman throwing his net into the water. Jesus approaches the man and says, "How long are you going to be a fisherman? Day in and day out, just catching fish? Perhaps there is more to your life than just this?" The fisherman responded that he had never really questioned it, but he could see that there must be more to life than just fishing. Jesus said, "If you come with me, I will teach you how to catch the hearts of men, to catch the beauty in humanity, rather than just catching fish." The fisherman obviously saw a depth, love, and sincerity in the eyes of Jesus that made the man unable to doubt him. The aura of stillness and calm that surrounded Jesus left the fisherman no choice but to hang up his net and follow Jesus into a fresh new destiny.

We can convince ourselves that we need to keep our identities as we know them intact. We think we need the stuff, the money, the status, the security, the big house, the persona we've created. Psychologist Carl Jung spoke openly about his lifelong desire to go to Rome to study the great written works within the Vatican library. For many years, he would periodically make train reservations and then cancel them. Though he longed to read these great works, at the same time he was afraid because he feared he would see in the great spiritual writings and works of the wise men of old that his life's work was all wrong. Jung was very honest about his conflicted feelings. It was as if a voice within him whispered, "What if I've built my whole life on sand? What will that say about my thought systems, my achievements, my identity?" Unfortunately, Jung never was able to step out of his comfort zone to make the journey to Rome because he so feared seeing himself in this new light.

At some level, we all have this conflict within us, and it scares us. We are afraid to let go, to face the groundlessness and uncertainty. Way down deep, we feel that if people saw the unmasked us, the naked us, the authentic us, they would recoil in horror. We are terrified of ourselves, so we

maintain the illusions, patch the leaks, and hide. We have become so very sophisticated at presenting our masks that we almost fool ourselves, but not quite. Many of us sense that something is wrong and that deep change is needed—a brave unveiling of who we are at our core. But we doubt ourselves and our worth, so, like Jung, at some level we cling to what already know and accept as reality. We veer away from taking that journey inward and therefore out of our comfort zone, not realizing that *the way out is in.*

Once we've gone inward, we can then step out beyond our comfort zone and find the courage to flow from our hearts. Going out on the ledge of our existence, we have no choice but to be real. When you are standing directly in the face of the unknown, all the rest of the phony stuff doesn't matter. In moments of great fear, everything else just falls away and there is nothing but you, your heartbeat, and your breath. Those are moments of pure truth, when you are cornered into simply *being.*

We cannot transform without leaving our comfort zone; there is no secret passage around this basic law. You must face your fears, relax in unconditional openness, and cut through all your tendencies to hold on. Jesus gave a talk one day to a group of his enthusiastic followers. He taught about the impermanence of all things and that nothing in life, including us, is solid or predictable. He told his students that any intellectual construct of reality was a noose that would get tighter and tighter and could only create suffering; so we must let go of everything and hold on to nothing so that virtue can shine through.

It can be tempting to keep our masks firmly in place, maintain the status quo, and hold firmly to the boundaries of our comfort zone. Yet as Jesus taught, life is about letting go of anything and everything that blocks wisdom from shining through.

Law 4: Commit to Growth

He turns not back who is bound to a star.

—LEONARDO DA VINCI

THERE IS AN ANCIENT NATIVE AMERICAN TEACHING THAT SAYS THAT WITHIN US ARE TWO WOLVES, WHICHEVER ONE WE FEED, WE STRENGTHEN. WITHIN EACH OF us, there exist two forces: a pull toward security—preservation of ourselves as we are—and a pull toward growth. Whichever we hold as more precious, we cultivate.

Growth requires a certain singleness of mind. As Jesus once said, "You cannot serve two masters." Either you commit to a change of heart and mind and live it out, or you are just playing around. This singleness of mind I'm talking about means making a total commitment to the path of growth: no wavering, no detours, absolute commitment to staying present, unconditional commitment to discovering and living by the truth within. I'm talking about staying the course, even when it hurts.

I once had a teacher who would refer to me as "undisciplined Baron." I lacked any sense of commitment, except to my own self-serving needs. Even in moments when I intuitively knew what was right, I would drown out my inner voice of conscience and essentially do whatever I wanted to do. If there was pleasure and something felt good, I went there. If something was uncomfortable or meant facing my self-centeredness, I was out of there. For me, the temptation to follow my feelings was a wonderful diversion, the perfect exit door from any kind of personal focus.

Never making a decision is a decision unto itself. It is a decision to stay in a personal fog. Staying in the confusion is safe, because in the fog, we never have to face the mundane that comes with committing to a path. Everyone tries to avoid the mundane path, but that is the path that makes us grow.

Many of us who have been married know the challenges that can come up. We decide, "Yes, this is the person I will spend the rest of my life with," and at some point, we start to see annoying habits and dark characteristics that we didn't notice before. The person who seemed so right is now the wrong one. We panic once we seal off the escape route, suddenly questioning whether we can, in fact, face this person each day. We can't see that very often the "wrong" person can actually be the right person, because he or she shows us parts of ourselves that need to be seen and healed. The real question might be "Can I face the parts of *myself* that this person dredges up in me each day?" Rather than learning this lesson, we take the nearest escape hatch as soon as things get uncomfortable. Of course, we eventually find out that if we don't learn our lessons through one vehicle, we will eventually have to learn them through another.

Ideally, we learn about staying rather than darting when we feel frustrated or threatened. If we are open enough, we can see how we have wanted love on our terms, and just in case it isn't delivered that way, we keep an exit door open. Very few of us would ever find ourselves in a situation that doesn't have at least one secret little exit door, a place where we can sneak through and out if we have to.

Each year I conduct a weeklong bootcamp in the mountains of Montana. A Lakota elder medicine man takes us through a sweat lodge ceremony, in which up to ten of us sit close together in a pitch-dark tent around a blazing fire, praying and chanting. I always notice an interesting phenomenon: Certain people insist on sitting right by the little exit flap of the tent. They are adamant, claiming they *must* be near the door. I have witnessed these same people break down into intense emotions, fear, and often racking sobs. You later hear them say that as the steam and heat increased and filled the space with full intensity, they were sure that something terrible was going to happen. They convinced themselves to stay by saying that if they were near the door, they would be able to make it through to the end. The truth is that even if they didn't sit by the door, they would make it through.

In our total commitment to inner revolution and growth, we don't get to sit near the door. We don't get to duck out if the process becomes uncomfortable. We learn to stay with ourselves, no matter what.

Eventually we are naturally ready to close our exit doors because we see that keeping them open is playing small in the big picture. The cool thing about this is that when we are truly committed to staying, we will know when and if it's *really* time to go.

So many of us lack commitment because we want to stay open to alternatives, to better sights than we see, better sounds than we hear, a better relationship than we are in. A student of mine in his thirties is very good-looking and continually dates one woman after another, each time eventually leaving his current relationship in pursuit of something better. He never stays long enough to fully get that the women are not the problem. In his mind, there will always be someone else out there who is prettier, sexier, smarter, funnier. By feeding the insatiable, self-centered wolf that craves the hunt, he essentially starves the wolf that would ultimately lead him to emotional maturity and spiritual fulfillment.

In our spiritual practice, we learn that even if every inch of our being wants to run in the opposite direction, we stay. These practices, at their core, are the art of staying. When we practice yoga and meditation, when we practice staying clear and conscious around food, or when we stay conscious of our reactions in all our relationships, we are strengthening our ability to be steadfast with ourselves. We are in a

discipleship. The word *disciple* comes from the same root as *discipline*. To be a disciple of your revolution means to be committed fully to doing the right thing, learning the lessons, and being open to the whole range of experiences that arise along the path. No matter what comes up—bone-aching emptiness, anger, or the craziest thoughts and emotions—we learn to stay right where we are.

One aspect of commitment is staying in our body. Although many yoga practitioners are tempted, we don't run out of the room during our practice if it gets challenging. We acknowledge the impulse to run as just another thought and let it go, without judging it or getting swept into the story of it. This is no small task. We have been thoroughly conditioned to bolt when we are uncomfortable, but we stay anyway, because this is how we awaken the sacred within us.

Are you experiencing cravings? Instead of reaching out, just stay with them. Is anxiety rising? Stay. Are fear and anger out of control? Stay. Are your muscles quaking, are you running out of steam? Stay anyway. Are your hips screaming in pigeon pose? Okay, but stay. We are the only ones who know and hear our internal dialogues, and we are the only ones who can make the choice to stay and unfold. Almost always, there is a breakthrough waiting for you right over the horizon.

Like every revolutionary throughout

history, you may stumble over rocks in your path that may make you want to give up. But through commitment, those rocks will cease to serve as roadblocks and begin to serve as potential points of new awareness. If you can call your conflicts and

troubles lessons, and remember that every experience develops some latent force within you, you will grow vigorous and happy, however adverse your circumstances may be.

Law 5: Shift Your Vision

Things don't change; we change.

—HENRY DAVID THOREAU

THE TIBETAN TANTRIC TEACHINGS SPEAK OF THE "SHIVANETRA," WHICH IS CONSIDERED THE EYE OF SHIVA, THE GREAT DEITY OF DESTRUCTION AND REGENERATION.

The Tibetans believe that between our two eyes is a third eye, which takes form inside our heads as the pineal gland. This third eye is the source of our spiritual vision. They teach that although this third eye exists in all of us, in most it is nonfunctioning. Through spiritual practice it begins to activate and open.

If we have had an opening and cleansing of the heart, the right energy can be released and spark life in this spiritual eye. If we pay attention to living according to our higher mind and our morals, it is said that this eye comes to life. As it awakens, so does our spiritual vision, and we begin to see ourselves and the world through new eyes.

Whatever spiritual or physical transformation process we are going through, we are seeking to undo and unlearn a thought system that has blinded our true vision. In life we run into obstacles that upon first glance *look* like the fault of others, but a closer examination will often show that the obstacles can be a mirror of our own hidden barriers. Every time we find ourselves in conflict, we immediately launch into the blindness of resentment and fear. We lose our eye of intuition and lose sight of what is real.

Yes and no are present in all things. To say yes to one thing automatically means saying no to another. If you do something wrong—if you hurt, you lie, you abuse—you are saying no to what's right. Saying yes to conscience and spirit is saying no to ego. Ultimately, through right intention, we have the power to say no to the ego and look through the lens of higher consciousness. To shift our vision means looking at the usual things with fresh eyes. As we start to spiritually awaken, our new vision allows us to see that most of our obstacles are created within our own hearts.

Our greatest power to change ourselves is found in our ability to see beyond the veil, to see with an enlightened vision. One of my oldest and best friends, Jesse, is a world-renowned public speaker. He has a daily radio show and has spoken in front of many influential organizations, including the United Nations. What very few people know is that in childhood Jesse suffered from a speech impediment. But Jesse is a man of faith. He so deeply and passionately believed in his message that he ignored the impediment and set his vision on getting the word out to as many people as he possibly could. Though he struggled and was ridiculed, his drive and belief were infectious, and doors opened to him despite his handicap. As the years went by, the intensity of his vision grew brighter, and his speech impediment fell away.

A vision shift calls for *attention, intention,* and *faith.* Attention is mental focus, and attention begets energy. Whatever you give your positive or negative attention to, you will energize, for better or for worse: a child, your body, a handicap. If you bring your attention to any point of your anatomy, you energize that point. Whatever you focus on, you fortify. Conversely, whatever you ignore will atrophy. If Jesse had lacked faith and dwelled on his handicap, chances are it would have worsened. But because he channeled his attention toward his true calling, his handicap withered away, and he was able to rightly influence the world.

Intention has tremendous power, because when you hold an awareness of what you need to do in the back of your mind, you direct your energy and the energy of the universe in that direction. As Ralph Waldo Emerson once said, "Once you make a decision, the universe conspires to make it happen." Intention sparks a recreation of events, and circumstances begin to organize toward their own fulfillment. Right intention leads us to the realm of flow, or what the Indians call *vinyasa.* When we find the pureness of our intention, we unleash a force that has the miraculous and infinite ability to rally circumstances, energy, situations, synchronicity, and serendipity all on our behalf. It's like trying to bake a cake. You need all the right ingredients, but you also need the right temperature for the right duration of time. The pieces all need to fall into place.

There is a danger to the phenomenal power of intention, however. If we use it for selfish purposes, to fulfill the insatiable appetite of our greedy ego, we fall out of alignment with the natural laws of right action and are heading for darkness. We have all read the stories in the news about the demise of greedy captains of industry who focus their intent on selfish gain and profit at the expense of others, or about politicians who abuse their power to further their own personal agendas. This is why we need what I call "right intent." In other words, intention is appropriate as long as you do not use it to violate the basic spiritual laws of goodness. Through right intent and a true repentance of the heart, you can transform your body, your life, and your world.

How can you know if an intent is from your pure heart? If you can honestly look at yourself in the cosmic mirror and feel at ease with your conscience, then it is pure. If it isn't, your conscience will signal you, loud and clear. However, we are so skilled at ignoring our conscience that it requires a real shift on our part to be open to it and hear it. You can blot it out and ignore it, but if you try to fool your conscience, it will make a fool out of you.

I often see students misuse healthy practices such as yoga in this way. They say their intention is to awaken, but really, their intention is to maintain the status quo of their ego. Whether they come to class because they want to have a better body, dissolve stress, or feed their competitive drive for accomplishment, they haven't looked at themselves in the mirror and *really* gone inward in order to spark an outward transformation.

A shift in vision also calls for faith. We get so caught up in things such as whether or not Moses really parted the Red Sea or if Jesus really rose from the dead, but the facts of these miracles are irrelevant. There is a certain leap of faith that we need to take. The real phenomenon is in our consciousness, in the power of what's possible. We don't necessarily need to know if Moses literally led the Jews through the desert to freedom or if Jesus emerged from the dead. We only need to trust that such transformation within humanity is possible. It is important that we don't just believe in it as an intellectual construct, but that we develop a heart of faith and use it as a great tool to shift from seeing with our literal eyes to seeing with our spiritual ones.

Law 6: Drop What You Know

Relinquishing control is the ultimate challenge of the spiritual warrior.

—THE BOOK OF RUNES

WHEN I TRAIN NEW YOGA TEACHERS, I USUALLY COME TO THE POINT WITH THEM WHERE I TELL THEM TO STOP STUDYING YOGA, STOP READING BOOKS ON PERSONAL

growth, stop going to workshops—simply stop looking to the outside for knowledge. The truth is that we reach a moment where we've read the books, done the workshops, followed this teacher or that one, and then we need to just *be the change*. More education is not always the solution. What is needed is a special kind of awakening that brings you to understand things for yourself. Dropping your brain means to rediscover, trust, and grow from this blessed state—which the ancient ones called *living by faith*.

Many years ago I had an experience while teaching a class in which I suddenly became aware of standing in front of the class speaking and having a consciousness separate from the words I was saying. Essentially, I was on automatic pilot. I noticed my words were just sounds that I was uttering and that I had no real connection to them. I was just regurgitating what I had read or heard other teachers say; nothing was flowing from my own experience and intuitive sense. As I stood back and listened to the language that was flowing out of my mouth, I actually felt stupid and awkward. In that moment, it was as though I knew nothing at all except the words I was delivering by rote. I realized I was completely dependent on learned knowledge to look and sound smart. I saw what a game that was, and how, because I had put so much faith in the words of others, I had no confidence and belief in my own ability to see, speak, and flow from the wordless language of my own heart.

This experience became a huge revelation to me. I began to really listen to the words that came out of me, but also the words that were floating around in my head. Were they my own? How about all the negative, self-defeating words and thoughts? Were they really me? I saw that the words of others (parents, peers, teachers, experts) directed my whole life and therefore in no way could I live authentically. I was robotically doing what the "knowledge" in my head said—I did yoga poses the way they were supposed to be done, ate the way I was supposed to eat. I was doing all the right things, but in a mechanical way that was devoid of my own intuition and common sense.

This inquiry lead me to that first humbling truth—that I didn't *really* know anything, and nothing that I could learn from rote would be worth anything real until it filtered down from my head into my heart and crystallized as a real part of me. I could learn and regurgitate all the intellectual constructs that I liked, but it wasn't until I was okay with not knowing that I began to really intuitively know things. Dropping my brain was the willingness on my part to drop all that I thought I knew, so that I could listen to something more profound within.

At a certain point we all need to make the shift from living from our head into trusting what's in our heart. We need to become intuitive beings. This is not easy. We have a lot invested in our knowledge base, including our identity and self-image. When we first start living from our intuition we feel clumsy and self-conscious, maybe even dumb, because we have to give up our learned "smartness." The truth is that whenever we start anything new, we will be awkward at it. It's like starting a new relationship—the first date is always awkward, but the more time you spend with that person the more familiar and comfortable he or she becomes to you, until one day there is more trust and a sense of certainty.

When I was growing up, my parents were yoga teachers who owned the largest health food store in San Francisco. Back then yoga and health food were still considered weird, and so I was teased a lot. The kids at school and in the neighborhood would call me "Hare Krishna." I remember the cruel chants about me and my family the kids would sing on the bus ride to school. Sometimes I would come home crying and tell my mother what they'd said. She would ask if what they said was true, and I would reply that it wasn't. She would always say, "Stick and stones may break your bones, but words can never hurt you—unless you empower them."

For many of us, throughout our school years, this sensitivity to words continued to shape us in ways we didn't even realize. Often in boring classrooms we were bombarded with dry, mechanical facts that were painful to memorize and devoid of meaning for us personally. Little or no attention was given to our true interests and talents. Many of us weren't allowed to discover things for ourselves. The idea was drilled into us that the sentences and ideas in the books are what is right and real. Too often, many of our educators lost sight of the fact the root of the word *education* is *educere,* which means "to draw forth from within." As a result, even to this day we are too easily influenced by what other people say. Praise makes us feel good, while criticism makes us feel bad. Even the tone of someone's speech has a way of getting under our skin. This oversensitivity to other people's words has an insidious way of eroding our faith in our own perceptions.

When I teach I often tell the class not to get caught up in the hypnosis of the group dynamic or in my words. I witness how quickly people lose themselves in what I say, and pretty soon they are not listening to themselves, their body, and what is right for them in each moment. So I remind them, "We live life from our heads, but here in this practice let's drop our brain and lead with our heart. The present mo-

ment has the opportunity for a rebirth. Forget the paradigms of the past, forget what all your teachers have told you—let's find out what the inner teacher has to say." Staying in our body and not in our head is a constant practice.

The ego thinks, "If I don't arm myself with an arsenal of knowledge, I will be inadequate, boring, and unprepared. I won't grow. I won't know what to do or say, or worse, I won't do or say it right." So we become dependent on outside knowledge; it becomes a crutch for us. It becomes a compensation for true wisdom. As long as we don't drop our brains, we will never have to make that internal shift to living from our center of conscience. The object, however, is to get ourselves and our stinking thinking out of the way so that we can wake up and grow.

There was a new student who came to a weekend workshop in northern California. Every time I asked if there were any questions, she would raise her hand and ask a question about the mechanics of yoga— why it works, what it does for us specifically, and how exactly it affects us. She wanted to know how the science of yoga worked; she wanted it all explained so that she could do it *right.* To each question, I suggested that she just go through the practice and let the experience speak for itself.

In every practice, though, she kept stopping to see if she was doing the poses right, continually lifting her head up and looking around. During the final day, I noticed that she seemed to have stopped trying to figure it all out and was flowing with the present moment's experience. At the end of the workshop, she came up to me, gave me a huge hug, and said, "Wow, something clicked in me. As soon as I stopped being absorbed in worry and doubt and whether I was doing it right, something in me shifted. I came out of my head and was able to let go."

We need to cast out our self-doubt. When we *really* let go, as this student did, suddenly we open up and there is space for new energy and insight; we go from myopic mind to big mind. Giving up our need to know and to be right creates space for life to unfold. "Not knowing" breaks us out of our old paradigms, our need to control and think our way through everything. There is such wisdom and healing power in not knowing. The paradox is that if we are really willing to not-know, we will. If you are in the now, you will always know how. You don't need to be an expert to understand this process. It's not intellectual; it's spiritual.

Faith is required if we are to let go of our "all-knowing" minds and dive into the realm of not-knowing. It is very empowering to be able to say "I don't know." What did Moses do when he found himself stuck between the Red Sea and Pharaoh's magnificent and vicious army? He admit-

ted he did not know what to do, and asked God for help. God told him to raise his staff, and a safe passage was created. Moses was literally stuck between the devil and the deep blue sea, and though many of those around him doubted and called him a failure and fraud, he had full trust in the power of God within him. Any logical brain would say that parting a sea is impossible, but when we silence that logic and rely instead on our faith in a force greater than us, miracles can happen.

When you stop thinking, you can come out of your head and become fully present in your body. It means noticing your doubts and then letting them go, endlessly releasing the thoughts and internal stories that reinforce your mental status quo. By letting go of your story line, you open the lines of communication between you and your higher power.

Don't analyze the process of transformation. We don't change by thinking; we change by *being* and *doing with a pure intent*. There is a story about two men, one a professor of philosophy, the other a sannyasin (seeker of truth), who were lost in the forest on a dark stormy night. The sounds of wild animals were chilling and the darkness dense. The storm grew stronger, the thunder louder, and suddenly lightning lit up the sky like the midday sun. The professor was looking up into the sky, watching the lightning and intensely analyzing their situation, and he didn't see the path through the forest, which was lit up in that moment. The sannyasin was watching the path and thus saw the way home.

When we are stuck in our heads, we are caught in a forest as dark as the one in the story. When a flash of lighting comes and lights the way, we must look for the light on our path so that we can take the right direction in that moment and go to new places in our lives. If you are reading about the forest, studying the map, or looking to me, the teacher, you miss out, because the lightning will not continue and darkness will return. The sannyasin knows that the lightning lasts only for a moment and that we must be fully present and open in order to see what it illuminates.

Law 7: Relax with What Is

Adversity reveals genius.

—HORACE

LIFE IS FULL OF PRESSURE AND DIFFICULT MOMENTS. IN AN INSTANT, WE CAN TURN THE ARROWS OF STRIFE INTO OPPORTUNITIES FOR PROFOUND CHANGE IF WE

simply learn to relax with what is. Wisdom comes from not losing our cool in turbulent moments. The yoga master B. K. S. Iyengar once said: "Before we can find peace among nations, we have to find peace inside that small nation which is our own being."

Years ago, I was leading a bootcamp in Hawaii. I was swimming in the ocean when all of a sudden a sea snake zipped through the water and latched onto the leg of a woman standing on the reef. She started screaming and screaming and screaming. I didn't have time to panic. I just reached down into the water, grabbed the snake, pulled it off her leg, and threw it far off into the distance. Something in me clicked, and I relaxed in that strange moment rather than flailing and freaking out. Because I was at ease, I was able to think on my feet and intuitively knew what to do.

Many of us have had moments like these. They serve as a powerful reminder that when we relax in the face of stress, a power greater than ourselves can act through us. At any given moment, the compassionate, frictionless flow of the universe wants to help us, if only we will allow it. We can always put our thoughts, our effort, our resistance, our reaction aside and trust in an intelligence that is, perhaps, smarter than we are.

Sometimes people ask me why my power yoga classes are so challenging. I've learned that intense physical challenge allows students to see in the moment how much more effective relaxing is than struggling. It's about bypassing your resistance. When you are at your most tired, you don't have the energy to resist. You relax, you stop forcing, essentially because there is no other choice, and then suddenly you discover that the source of grace was there waiting for you all along, willing and happy to help you discover a strength and wisdom that you in fact already have. The moment you stop forcing a result, you develop a mental and muscular poise under pressure.

For instance, hip-opening poses can feel very intense, because we hold not only gravity but also our emotional lives in our hips. As the pressure builds, you are faced with three choices: (1) run away (i.e., come out of the pose), (2) stay and struggle, or (3) stay, relax, and discover what is really there.

I have a student who is a writer and sits in a chair for long hours every day, making her hips especially tight. She shared with me an experience she had during a practice: She was getting tired and just didn't have the energy to struggle and resist any longer, so she let go of her mental rope and relaxed into her body. When she relaxed, the physical pain was much less, and revelations began to explode in her mind. What started as a struggle became a spiritual experience for her. All through that long hold, she would ask herself, "Is there another level I can relax into . . . another layer I can surrender into?" The answer each time was yes, and in the end her hip joints relaxed and flowered open to a whole new degree, as did her self-perception.

In this release, she saw her practice as a microcosm of her whole life. She acknowledged that she had an unconscious fear that if she let go, she would see how out of control she actually was in her life, and how much of this stemmed from a deeper sense of insecurity. Deep down, she believed that if anyone saw how she *really* was, they would reject her, so she held on tightly to the mask she'd created. Without realizing it, many of us find a way to keep our own natural peace at bay, and control is certainly one means of doing so. Ideally our practice shows us how to transform difficult circumstances into a path of enlightenment.

In yoga practice, there may be sensations that you don't like, and that's okay. Don't judge. Simply realize that pain is part of life. If you grow, there is pain, and if you *don't* grow, there is pain. The key is in noticing and *not* reacting. Of course, you will want to make the distinction between good and bad pain. If it is bad pain, which will feel sharp and electric, your body is sending you a message to back off. Good pain, on the other hand, feels more like a deep stretch, a soreness, or a strong sensation in your muscles; this is the threshold to a new body, a new psychology, and a new spirit. As uncomfortable as it is, it usually holds lessons and can give new direction if we stay open and relax with the discomfort *just as it is.*

Law 8: Remove the Rocks

The block of granite which was an obstacle in the path of the weak
becomes a stepping stone in the path of the strong.

—THOMAS CARLYLE

TRANSFORMATION MEANS REMOVING THE ROCKS FROM OUR GARDEN, THE BOULDERS THAT BLOCK OUR NATURALNESS. THE PRACTICES IN THIS BOOK ARE NOT SO

much a learning process as an unlearning process. We unlearn our pride, our anger, our fear, our conditioning, and our resistance and come back to our natural way of being. When we were kids, we were free and innocent. As time passed, we accumulated the rocks of resistance, piling them up until they become mountains in our minds.

Transformation comes not by adding things on but by removing what didn't belong in the first place. We change by peeling away all the toxic layers, emotional debris, and beliefs that we have added on over the years. We forget that there is

something perfect already within us; through years of habit and hypnosis we took a wrong turn, and now we automatically look outside ourselves for something that will fix us.

In and of themselves, the practices in this book do nothing. The yoga does nothing, the meditation does nothing, the self-awareness exercises do nothing, balancing your diet does nothing. Neither I nor any other teacher can give you a magic cure. "Wait a second," you might be thinking. "Then why should I do these things?" Because they are a road map back to your center, back to your inner teacher: your conscience. The techniques are the way to the way, but they are not the end in themselves; they do not possess any power of their own. They are simply tools for excavation. We think that we have struggles and problems in life, but the only problem we have is a disconnection from our center. When we come back to self, all the other things begin to take care of themselves, and our lives begin to flow.

Baptiste Power Vinyasa Yoga rinses out toxins, peels away layers of tension, and helps to clear away the heaviness we hold trapped in our body. The poses can break down the painful but familiar holding patterns and return us to our natural body. And when patterns are broken, new worlds emerge.

We remove the clutter from our minds through meditation. It enables us to keep ourselves clear, like an open vessel, to let the wisdom and light flow through. I believe awareness-based meditation is the single most powerful tool for transformation. The greatest power we have over ourselves is our ability to change our minds about ourselves. By quieting our minds, we travel directly into the center of our mental cyclone to a clearer place of deep knowing and spiritual understanding. This calm wisdom within is always there; it is part of our nature that we have obscured. On a cloudy day, the sun is not absent; it is just blocked by the clouds. Meditation burns away the clouds and lets the sun-

shine of truth come through. In time, through practice, we begin to notice the clouds as just passing things rather than permanent obstructions.

It's as if Publishers Clearing House was trying to call and tell you that you'd won the grand prize, but you were on the phone and all they were getting was a busy signal. Unless you stop chatting and let the line go free, you aren't able to receive the bounty and great gift that awaits you. Meditation is like putting up your antennae to receive that signal. When you put the noise and chatter aside, you can receive the insight, the wisdom, and the greater message of the universe struggling to come through to you.

The excavation questions in this program can dig up the rocks in your mind and give you insight into your trigger points. To the degree that we are willing to see clearly our self-destructive patterns, they lose their hold on us and wither away. There is tremendous power in just knowing what is going on within us, not so that we can "work on our stuff," but so that we can begin to release it. Many of us spend much of our lives wrapped up in the drama of our stories. We become very adept at knowing all about our problems, but the key is not to stop there. The key is to see beyond pathology into an enlightened vision.

When I was living in Los Angeles, I used to know a woman who was overweight and who was fixated on losing her extra twenty-five pounds. She went to every diet doctor in town and tried every sure-thing program out there. Atkins, The Zone, Weight Watchers—you name it, she did it. She spent thousands of dollars going to a therapist to talk about her binge eating, and she could talk all about how and when she overate. Yet for all her efforts, never once did she stop to actually look past the symptoms (overweight) or the habits (overeating). She wasn't able to see and heal the deeper source of pain in her heart that was being masked.

This woman attended a weekend work-shop, and a few weeks later, I received a letter from her. It said:

Dear Baron,

At the retreat earlier this month, you were talking about the principle of removing our rocks, and I had this huge shift in perspective. I realized I have my own personal rock collection, and those rocks are grinding against my heart and creating dust in the form of anxiety, depression, doubt, and regret. The rocks are all the moments that my mother told me I couldn't do anything right: that I wasn't talented enough, smart enough, or pretty enough. I now see how I was living a self-fulfilling prophesy. I was looking for things to fail at, like a diet, because if I continued to fail, I would prove that my mother's perceptions of me were right. But all I was really doing was

avoiding the deeper issue, which is this sense of worthlessness I've been carrying around with me all these years.

I finally saw that only through softening my heart and forgiving would I heal the unfinished business with my mother, which was ultimately the real excess weight I was carrying around.

I see hints of the same phenomenon the first night of every bootcamp, when we go around the room and everyone says aloud the one thing he or she wants to let go of that week. There are always a few people who say things like "my love handles," or "Oreo cookies" or "cigarettes." That first night, they truly believe that their love handles or the cookies or the cigarettes are the problem. As the week goes by they usually come to a sense of clarity and natu-ralness, and they begin making shifts in perspective that reach way beyond the sur-face struggles. They begin to see what the behaviors were masking.

Plato speaks about the shadow behind things. It is as though life is a wheel and all the aspects of our lives are the spokes of the wheel. At the center of this wheel is the source, a miraculous force from which we take our energy. We get caught up in the spokes—the delusions and projections—and lose our connection to the center. But by coming back to center, we can reach into the shadows and direct life from the cause. It is so important for us to get that we don't have to solve any of our problems. If we can soften our heart, give up some of our old ways of being, and reconnect to the truth, our problems will give us up.

The journey of transformation is always a journey back to the center of truth, and once we reach that center, the rocks that clutter our minds begin to disintegrate.

What rocks are you holding on to?

Law 9: Don't Rush the Process

Have patience with all things, but chiefly have patience with yourself.
Do not lose courage in considering your own imperfections,
but instantly set about remedying them—every day begin the task anew.

—SAINT FRANCIS DE SALES

THERE IS A BIBLICAL SAYING, "LORD, PLEASE SHOW US THE SHORTNESS OF DAYS SO THAT WE MIGHT HAVE WISDOM OF HEART." LIFE IS SHORT. AT SOME LEVEL WE ALL KNOW that, and so we rush to complete all that we think we must do in order to live a life of no regrets. We get swept up in our accomplishing, doing, and achieving so completely that we miss out on the natural order of unfolding, and anguish and tremendous imbalance are the result. In our impatience, we create the very scenario that we hoped to avoid. Jesus asked, "What good will it be for a man if he gains the whole world, yet forfeits his soul?"

Through patience, you can possess your soul. When you catch yourself speed-ing through life, when you feel you must meet expectations and that so much is be-ing left undone or that you're not succeed-ing as quickly as you think you should be, you must remember that real growth doesn't come from pushing through or breaking out of anything. Rather, it comes through a gentle melting in. The path of patience asks you to be okay with what is, stare it straight in the eye, and open to and learn from what's happening rather than contracting into fear, frustration, and a hidden drive to meet your expectations at any costs. We must remember that when

34

everything has to be right, something usually isn't.

There is a silly Zen saying, "Don't just do something, sit there," but there is a lot of wisdom in that, too. When we're confronted with our own impatience as well as another's, we can sit there and create the space for the usual habitual pattern *not* to happen. Through the practice of patience we increase the gap between stimulus and response; we learn to be okay with our restlessness and our sense of guilt about not doing enough, and then we can hopefully begin to let these things go.

Patience does not mean that we resign ourselves to a situation and just endure it. Instead, we can stop resisting and open to something better and take right action. Over the years, I have had interns come to work for my institute, and there is always a clear division between two types of attitude. The first attitude occurs in the ones who are impatient to advance, who resent the menial work. They want to run before they crawl. They want to get ahead quickly, but they are resisting where they are, and thus there is an energy block. The second attitude occurs in the ones who have a love for the work, who want to absorb everything at the level where they are. They are willing to be patient with their growth within the process, and their work flows easily and joyfully as a result. If we are so wound up in getting somewhere, we

don't realize that every step of the way, we missed where we were. The irony of personal growth is that when we slow down and fully engage in the present, we usually get to where we *really* want to go faster.

At a teacher training bootcamp, we had about a hundred students who were there to learn how to teach Baptiste Power Vinyasa Yoga. Some of the students were struggling with the essence of being present with a roomful of people and teaching the sequence of postures all at once. They were getting upset with themselves for fumbling or forgetting the poses. Finally, a student told a story about her personal progress as a teacher. She said, "I learned I had to be willing to show up and suck until I could show up and shine."

That became the mantra of the week, and from that moment forward, the energy shifted. For the most part, people could drop the anger toward themselves and were able to be okay with wherever they were in the process. In fact, there was a feeling of patience that radiated throughout the room. It was a joy to see.

Everything in life has a natural order and rhythm of unfolding that cannot be violated. If we force a rose to blossom, we break off its petals. If we pressure our kids to perform faster and place demands and schedules on them that are unnatural to who they are, their spirits are broken. Is it any wonder that so many of our kids end up on medication? Everything in nature has to grow in its sequential stages, and no stage can be skipped. A caterpillar goes into its cocoon before it emerges as a soaring butterfly. A seed is nurtured and simultaneously challenged to break out of its protective shell, then break through rocks and weeds out of the earth's crust, only to be met by the harshness of the sun, the abrasive nature of the wind and rain. It becomes a sprout, then eventually grows into a tree.

The principle of process is a law that our culture is constantly attempting to defy. It is a law that cannot be broken, however, so we end up breaking ourselves against it instead. For many of us it's easy to accept this law when we see it in nature, but personally we want to cheat it. We want the quick fix. We want to skip the vital steps, especially the steps that are uncomfortable or that scare us, so we look for shortcuts in order to save time and bypass discipline. We keep taking shortcuts until we realize that those paths were cheap or fleeting and that they eventually led us right back to where we were before.

The inner revolution of growth is about passing through fires. When I was working with the NFL, it was obvious that the coaches and players recognized that there is no shortcut to achieving skill. You need the commitment and calm determination to wait, to show up, to stay with it, even when it doesn't feel good. The very struggle of the process is what makes you sharp and gives you valuable experience and maturity. How can you achieve unconscious competence through a shortcut?

Many of us want the St. Paul experience of instantaneous wisdom and spiritual vision, the Buddhist satori of sudden enlightenment, but the small chunks and little shifts are just as valuable, because they are cumulative. The Zen masters say that a constant drip weares away a big rock. The greatest benefits come from the small shifts that move us into new directions.

A student experienced a wave of euphoria in class one day. In one instant, he suddenly "got it." Everything came into alignment for him in that one shining moment: the mistakes he was making in his life, his impatience with everything (including himself), and the deeper meaning of it all. Of course, he woke up the next day more frustrated than ever. "We get swept away pretty easily, don't we?" I said, and he nodded. A lot of people in the room smiled, because we've all had moments like these. These moments can feel like a tease, but they serve as a compass to show us where we want to be.

Our greatest source of wisdom is what is happening to us right now, where we are. But our rushing and pushing past the present moment cause us to miss out. In our efforts to do more and get wherever we want to go faster, we forget that we simply cannot rush the process and still expect to be *really* successful at anything. True growth is not cheap. Emotional maturity and seasoning come through an intimate understanding of the process of life, the love of the journey, and the depth of subtlety that is achieved through a commitment to patience.

Law 10: Be True to Yourself

The death of dogma is the birth of reality.

—IMMANUEL KANT

IN THE FAMOUS BIBLICAL STORY OF NOAH'S ARK, NOAH WAS ALREADY ALMOST FIVE HUN-DRED YEARS OLD WHEN HE HEARD THE VOICE OF GOD IN HIS HEAD commanding him to build a giant four-hundred-foot ark. Noah had never seen a boat in his lifetime, let alone a four-hundred-foot ark, so he certainly did not possess the knowledge of how to build such a thing. But he was guided by God's instructions, which came through him. The wicked people all around him laughed, but still Noah heeded his instinct to trust God and kept working. Though it took 120 years, Noah completed the ark, and as the parable goes, he, his family, and two members of every species were the only ones on earth saved from the floods that rushed forth. Had Noah not stayed true to himself, the world as we know it would have been made altogether extinct.

Being true to yourself means looking within to discover what you know in your heart to be right and then acting on it. It does not mean following every last whim or urge that you might have; that is just selfishness in disguise. It means being true to your values and morals. It means being honest in all things: knowing the truth, walking by that truth, and living by that truth. Regarding truth, Gandhi said:

What then is Truth? A difficult question, but I have solved it for myself by saying it is what the voice within tells you. How then, you ask, [do] different people think of different and contrary truths? . . . [I]t is because we have at the present moment everybody claiming the right of conscience without going through any discipline whatsoever that there is so much untruth being delivered to a bewildered world. All that I can in true humility present to you is that truth is not to be found by anybody who has not got an abundant sense of humility. If you would swim on the bosom of the ocean of Truth, you must reduce yourself to a zero.

Many of us have come to learn that when we live in alignment with the truth, our life works. We forget to treat that as something sacred. The word *sacred* tends to imply some pretty, untouchable thing—something that is beyond us. People go on pilgrimages to sacred places and take part in sacred rituals, and project all kinds of meaning onto them. But sacredness is really just the simplicity of living by our conscience, by our own intuitive light. The sacred is within us, of us, not *out there* somewhere. *Sacred* literally means "regarded with reverence," and ultimately, it is up to us what we choose to revere.

To be true to oneself means becoming a sannyasin, which in the East is a spiritual warrior—a seeker of truth and a revolutionary. Not necessarily a revolutionary involved in political revolution, but a revolution within oneself. The path of the sannyasin is a lonely one, because no one can do it for us. It is solitary because only we can remove what blocks the basic goodness, dignity, and wisdom within us. Gandhi, Socrates, Jesus: They were all sannyasins. Each sought the truth within and lived by it, come what may. As spiritual warriors, we must stand in our full worth, and we must honor what the sacred voice within tells us if we are to transform ourselves and the world around us.

Many of us have learned that in order to follow our inner compass and be true to ourselves, we have to be willing to go against the status quo. As a teacher, I believe my greatest power lies in my commitment to my own intuitive way of doing things, regardless of whether others approve or not. As a sannyasin, you, too, will need to find this in your own way. Transformation is the process of self-actualization, and self-actualizing people do not live at the mercy of forces outside of themselves.

It is not always easy to go against the grain. People unconsciously hate change, and those who cling to their hypnotic traditions are deeply attached to maintaining the "sacredness" of the status quo. If you think back throughout history, whenever a visionary emerges and says, "Hey, we have a better way!" those in the status quo crowd *never* say, "How great!" The status quo said to Jesus, "Who are you?" And they took this man who had healed and helped many people and hurt no one, and they killed him. Socrates had a beautiful, illumined spirit, and he loved interacting with people and expanding their thinking. He was accused of corrupting the Athenian youth, and the traditionalist leaders of the time poisoned him.

People such as Jesus, Socrates, and Gandhi threaten the status quo because they hit against our constellations, our patterns, our conditioning; they expose our reality, and that can be painful. But I always tell my students that the genuine transformational experience is *by its nature* disruptive of the existing state of affairs.

There was a time in my life when speaking my real truth was difficult for me. Back then, I needed the approval of others—my students, my teachers, my friends—to feel I was okay. I wouldn't speak my truth if I thought it would mean losing the approval I craved. But the real me underneath was full of knots, anxiety, and fear, because I was drawing my self-worth from a false source. I wasn't being true to anything, least of all myself.

In those days, I could not go against the crowd. If I did, I would come up against a strange energy within myself that felt very guilty and threatened, as if I were doing something wrong. To speak out in opposition felt like I was plunging a knife into my own heart. On the few occasions I actually did speak up, I would immediately start to doubt the validity of my own perception. Sometimes I would speak out and exclaim my truth, but in the wrong way: with anger, high emotion, and judgment. Ego speaks and ego listens, and my wrong expression would spark a wrong reaction in others. We would get all high on drama and judgment, and in the end, only our wounded pride was served.

At a certain point, through my own inner revolution, I started to wake up and become more objective in my own life. It was as though I had stepped out of a fishbowl and was now looking in as a witness. I found myself patiently standing outside the crowd within my own intuitive, protective bubble. Something within me was changing. Within this bubble I felt that I was growing and flowering into the real person I was meant to be. I could see a lot of the trancelike craziness that had overcome me in the past, and how I compulsively and blindly jumped for every bone of approval that was thrown my way.

As I got committed to the right source within me, I found a new self-confidence, and I learned to speak from my heart to the hearts of others. My knees would rattle, but each time I would speak directly from my own truth, great healing was occurring within me and I was being set free. I began to doubt my doubts, and started to find how to be true to myself in a more graceful way. I could disagree without being disagreeable, because I was no longer taking everything personally.

How does this apply to you and to your own process of transformation? Each and every time you say or do something that is completely true to you, regardless of what the status quo has to say about it, you access your greatest power and move closer to authentic whole-life health. What does this have to do with health? Everything, because we are either expressing or repressing, and if we are stuffing down, holding in, and repressing, then that energy will eventually manifest as disease. For instance, say that someone offends you and then later acts as if nothing happened. Should you allow that person to continue with a business-as-usual attitude toward you without apologizing? If you do, you surely must see that you are acting in subtle agreement with ignorance and falsity. At the very least, you will have blown your chance to clear the air and heal the situation. You might not have understood the other person's intent, and truly he or she might not have ever meant to offend you, but if you fail to speak your truth in a timely way, a cloud will continue to hang over the relationship and resentment will potentially percolate within you. Is that the truthful way to relate to a brother or sister? You need to constantly be on the alert to keep things clean. In this way of being, you are being true to yourself, and to others.

Law 11: Be Still and Know

Silence is a great help to a seeker of truth, like myself. In the attitude of silence, the soul finds the path in clearer light, and what is elusive and deceptive resolves itself into crystal clearness.

—GANDHI

IT IS OUR CHOICE: WE CAN SPEND OUR LIVES NURTURING RESENTMENTS AND HUNGERS, OR WE CAN VENTURE FORWARD AS WARRIORS OF LIGHT AND SEEKERS OF

truth, cultivating an open heart and real health. Many of us keep reinforcing our self-betraying habits and therefore keep fertilizing the seeds of our own suffering and failure. But through the practices that align us to the natural laws of life, we can instead sow the seeds of vitality and well-being. It begins with coming into stillness so that we may be able to know and understand the truth within.

Buddha came into being about twenty-five hundred years ago, and one of the things he did was describe how consciouness worked. He taught about the law of karma, cause and effect, action and reaction—how the energy you put out comes back to you. Five hundred years later, Jesus came along and taught that in a moment of grace, all your past actions are burned away like paper in a flame. If we keep overreacting to small things, we stay on our karmic wheel of suffering. Through the practice of coming into stillness, we can lift the level of our attitude and begin to respond in new ways, creating space for grace.

In the lower moments of my life, my humanness makes me feel vulnerable, fearful, and filled with doubt. Becoming still in meditation and prayer allows my higher power to come in and overtake the dark corners of my mind, lighting it with grace. Usually that means sitting quietly and sweating bullets if need be. When I say sit, I mean I simply close my eyes, open my mind, and relax with what is. When thoughts arise, I let them dissolve. If I do drift off, I simply begin again and again, coming back to that open, relaxed state of mind that bears witness to the moment at hand. Sometimes I center my attention on my hands, using them as an anchor, and sometimes I will just watch the naked ebb and flow of my breath. There is no manipulating the breath, just a bare-bones attentiveness to it, to my hands, and to a general sense of my surroundings. With my ears open, I use every sound as a reference point to the present moment. The practice is to stay present with the ordinary truth that arises in each moment and let it stand on its own, without building a story around it.

When you close your outward eyes, the energy starts moving backward and inward. Energy has to move somewhere; close one outlet and it will find another. Closing our physical eyes in meditation directs the energy to awaken within you. As the Old Testament says, "As the sensual eyes close, the spiritual eyes open." The yogis call this phenomenon *pratyahara*.

Voltaire said, "The most important decision we make each day is to be in a good mood." Meditation sets my mood. Usually upon arising, my mind calls me to immediately launch into my day, getting my kids off to school, getting dressed, checking messages, and making calls. At this point in my life, I know that this energetic pattern only contributes to mental chaos. If I've taken no steps toward establishing a change of heart within myself, then it will be no wonder that I'm feeling crazy and disconnected by midday.

The flip side is that if I set aside twenty to thirty minutes each morning for meditation and prayer and just quietly sit with myself, my experience of life becomes very different, because I'm different. By sitting still, my mind is renewed, and I anchor to something in me that can shine a light into my life. So before I do anything else, I've learned to commit to putting first things first. I anchor to self. I make the connection to conscience, putting on my spiritual armor before I head off into my day. Before I even take a step outside my door, I set myself right.

Each morning there is a war within me. My human side does not want to meditate and be still, but because of my commitment, my spiritual side wins in that moment. I've learned that laziness sabotages my inner life and undermines my confidence and self-respect. To sit requires more self-discipline, but the rewards are many.

In this sacred time, I can give my ego a hard time. Zen masters speak of meditation as the willingness to die over and over again. Jesus said, "I die daily." I believe this to mean that as we raise our consciousness, self-destructive attitudes die. Fears die. Resentments die. As the stuff of the ego dies through the act of melting into stillness, the spirit is born and we are renewed.

How does my morning meditation renew me? It definitely gives me a sense of humor. I used to say to myself: "I'll laugh about this situation five years from now." Now, I can stay light in difficult moments with more ease, because I know that if I can laugh about it in five years, I can laugh about it now. It also gives me the patience and peace to compassionately steer away from debilitating habitual patterns. I am brought into the present moment, and the present moment is the perfect teacher. I am less reactive and more calm in challenging moments.

I feel plugged into a basic sense of goodness that springs forth from within me, affecting the outcomes of situations in untold ways. I am more anchored to my conscience, which allows me to make good decisions with less confusion. My time spent in stillness gives feet to my prayers. This practice not only makes me feel better, but literally makes me a better person.

As with the beginning of my day, I also end my day with a period of stillness, to clean out the mental clutter I may have accumulated during the day so as to not take it

to bed with me. My sleep is sounder, cleaner, and more refreshing when the residue of my day isn't churning within me.

When I teach, I notice what a low tolerance people have for discomfort. I see so many students who will go to any means to avoid stillness. They go to great lengths to prevent themselves from moving closer to their feelings and emotions and getting in touch with their bodies. They fidget, fix their hair, take a drink of water, and leave to go to the bathroom, but I wonder—what if they stayed and simply dropped into stillness? What would they find there?

The truth is that a lot of us choose to stay busy and in a fog because we don't want to see and feel what is really there. But the truth will follow us and poke at us until we acknowledge it. Is there some tiny, dim awareness about yourself or your life that is lingering in the corners of your consciousness but which you try to ignore? We have become masters at drowning out that truth—that small, quiet voice within. This inner knowing whispers the way to live in our brightest light if we would only stop and stay still enough to listen, and then humble ourselves enough to follow.

The great philosopher Krishnamurti was asked, "Do we learn from experience?" His answer was, "No! We don't learn from experience. We learn what we *choose* to learn from experience." The time we carve out to spend in silence with ourselves and with God gives us the space in our mind to truly learn from experience.

Stillness is not only a thirty-minute exercise in the morning and at night. It is also a way of life—a gradual cessation of excessive busyness, planning, running around, accumulating, and stressing about things. Eventually, our aim is to have our inner stillness reflect outward into all the comings and goings of our lives.

Law 12: Understand That the Whole Is the Goal

In nature, the overall principles represent a higher reality than does the single object.

—ALBERT EINSTEIN

DURING A WORKSHOP I DID IN NEW YORK CITY, A WOMAN SHARED THAT SHE HAD READ *JOURNEY INTO POWER* AND HAD INCORPORATED A LOT OF THE PRINCIPLES AND practices from that book into her life. Her body was getting leaner and healthier through the yoga and the cleansing diet, but she was still filled with anxiety and was highly reactive in her relationships.

"Do you meditate?" I asked her.

"Well," she admitted, "I actually read the whole book except for that section."

"Then there's your answer!" I said. "Somehow you unconsciously avoided what you most needed."

We don't transform in parts. Every aspect of ourselves and our lives is interconnected with every other one. To paraphrase something Gandhi once said, "You cannot do wrong in one part of your life and expect to do right in all the others." There are some things that are known only in their wholeness, that you cannot dissect, and health is one of them. True health is not just an illness-free body, nor a peaceful and clear mind, nor clean eating or a higher purpose in life—it is all of those things combined, with a love of and a connection to your own conscience. Health is wholeness.

Aesop's fable of the goose and the golden egg is a wonderful example of how we become so fixated on the golden eggs rather than the bigger picture. We chase the treasures, so obsessed by the eggs of gold that we kill the goose that in fact gives us a life of true wealth. In our narrowed vision, we miss the point.

In the West, things are dissected into pieces. The self-help movement has fragmented the truth into many parts, from which we choose what we like and reject what we don't like. If you look at the various self-help books in the bookstore, you'll see they are usually broken down by category: a diet book over here, a health and fitness book over there, emotional and spiritual wellness books someplace else. Many of us take the pieces we like and obsess over them, usually abandoning the single-pronged path once it fails us, quickly moving on to another.

But true health is more than just the sum of the parts. If you dissect health, you miss it. If you dissect the truth, you miss it. If your goal is to have a toned body, chances are you will achieve that through the yoga practices in this book, but if that is your end goal, again, you're missing the bigger picture. It may be helpful to look at your life like a symphony: If you take apart the notes and sounds, one by one, you miss the magic of the music. It loses something, just as you do when you choose to work on only certain aspects of yourself rather than your whole being.

A revolution cannot be effective if it strives to change only bits and pieces of a society. Imagine if our forefathers had fought the British only for freedom of religion rather than total independence. Imagine if Martin Luther King Jr. had sought to change the transportation system in this country only so that the black American community could ride at the front of the bus, or if Gandhi had led the Indian people to fight merely for better living conditions rather than for full self-governing powers. Certainly they might have won these battles, but it was the overhaul of the entire system that led to sweeping and revolutionary changes.

The goal here is to make peace with all the tendrils and conflicts of your life, both inside and out, weaving the strands together into your own spiritual coat of many colors. In the end, if you dedicate your energies to detaching from struggle, giving up fear, taking right action, and practicing true patience within yourself, you will find that all the pieces of your life begin to radiate with the luminosity of whole and true health.

PART TWO

The Transformative Journey

40 Days to Personal Revolution

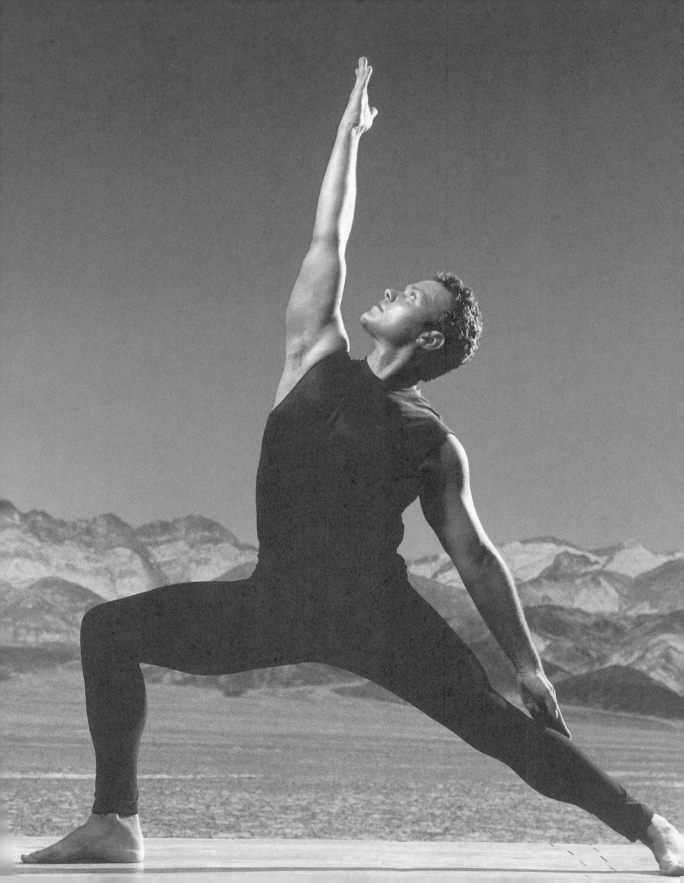

WITH THE LAWS OF TRANSFORMATION SERVING AS YOUR PHILOSOPHICAL FOUNDATION, YOU'RE READY TO BEGIN YOUR FORTY DAYS TO PERSONAL REVOLU-

tion. This introduction will give you a complete overview of the four different pieces of the program you will do each week—the daily yoga practice, diet insight and plan, meditation, and excavation questions. So once you get started, all you'll need to do is show up and flow.

Each week is centered on a theme, which will be the focus for your yoga and meditation practice, your new diet insight, and your excavation questions. Of course, forty days does not come out to exactly six weeks, but for the sake of clarity and ease, I have divided the progression into weeks, the last of which is only five days. The progression of the weeks corresponds to the arc of growth you will experience as you move through your forty days. The themes are:

Week One: Come into Your Body
Theme: Presence

Week Two: Fan the Purifying Flame
Theme: Vitality

Week Three: Be the Eye of the Hurricane
Theme: Equanimity

Week Four: Receive the Radiance
Theme: Restoration

Week Five: Root Down to Fly High
Theme: Centering

Week Six: Invite the Light
Theme: Triumph

Daily Yoga Practice

Really, at its heart, yoga is meant to be *physical* practice. Even the famous yogi Krishnamacharya said that asanas are designed for physical fitness. What we get here in the West are dressed-up practices that are infused with all kinds of Hindu undertones and religious ritual. But authentic yoga, as it is taught in India, is a physical practice that enables us to strengthen and free the body so that we may use it for greater purposes. It is the physical training of the sannyasin. Often the physical practice can calm the mind enough so that if the practitioner is ready, then perhaps spiritual insight may reveal itself.

Baptiste Power Vinyasa Yoga is a purposeful workout that will build a flexible and integrated strength, help rinse out toxins and dissolve tensions, and, if need be, release excess weight from your body, so that you can have a stable and balanced foundation from which to flow in life. Perhaps you already know from experience— and if not, you will discover—that Power Vinyasa Yoga practice sculpts and frees your natural body by removing what does not belong authentically. Finally, it creates a flexible strength and functional stability throughout your entire body.

The length of the practices will increase each week, starting with twenty minutes and working up to ninety. It is essential that you practice DAILY during these forty days, to hardwire the benefits into your nervous system. It is best to practice first thing in the morning, before eating, because your mind and body are free from clutter and therefore more impressionable than at any other time during the day. It is a wonderful way to set the tone of your day. Plus, if you don't get it in the morning, you very likely won't do it later as you get caught up in your day. The discipline of getting up just a little bit earlier each day will soon prove to be golden to you, as the power of the morning is invaluable.

Some days your practice may feel easy; other days it might feel next to impossible. It is important to realize that your practice is just what it is. Good or bad, up or down, just stay committed and don't judge it. Some days we flow, while other days we are stuck. I've breezed through practices, and I've also been through some in which all kinds of stuff has come up, including nausea and emotions, but I don't fret about it, because that is just what needs to happen.

You may be wondering whether you should continue your usual fitness activities. I would say you can continue, but I would also encourage you to lessen them. This program will give you what you need, and as you progress, you may no longer want to do your other activities. Just do the Power Vinyasa Yoga practice outlined here and let it create a foundation within you. After forty days, if you want to reintegrate cardio or weights, you can do so, and I'm sure you'll notice these will take on a whole new life. The way you move, the way you breathe, the way you focus—it will all be improved.

What You Will Need

The only thing you must have for your daily yoga practice is a sticky mat, which will prevent your feet from slipping (yoga is done barefoot) and provides padding. You can find one at almost any yoga studio or sporting goods store, or online. I sell the kind I like best on my Web site, www.baronbaptiste.com. If you want, you can use props such as yoga blocks, blankets, or straps to help you modify poses in the beginning stages.

Your Breath—the Key to Your Body's Potential

A master key of yoga practice is maintaining steady, rhythmic breath. Your breath is pure life force that regenerates you with every inhalation and cleanses you on every exhalation. Your breath links your mind to your body, and you to the present moment. It can and should carry you through your entire practice. By staying calm and breathing through your poses, the layers of resistance and tension dissolve and you can break through to new ground.

The breath we use in asana practice is called *ujjayi*. Ujjayi breathing is audible,

with a soothing, rhythmic quality. It is done by contracting the whispering muscles in your throat to create a long, hairline thin breath. You do not breathe all the way down into your abdomen, but rather into your chest, lungs, and back. If you breathe down into your belly, the power of ujjayi is lost.

Here is a step-by-step breakdown of how to do it:

1. Bring your first or second finger to the soft spot between your collarbones.
2. With your mouth closed, breathe in through your nose, contracting the whispering muscles in your throat. You should feel the gentle retraction of those muscles beneath your finger. You are closing the airway a little, so it is kind of like breathing through a straw.
3. For the exhalation, put your hand in front of your face as if it were a mirror. Gently retract your belly and, with your mouth closed and the muscles in your throat still contracted, exhale through your nose as if you were going to fog up that mirror. The exhalation should be exaggerated and extended.

Those are the basics of how you do it. The inhale and exhale should be equal in length and volume. In general, you inhale as you reach up and open in poses, and exhale as you fold down or close.

If you get dizzy, it probably means you

are forcing the breath too much. Though the ujjayi breath is exaggerated, it should also be relaxed and effortless. You don't want to take in too much or too little air; just let it be steady and free.

In Baptiste Power Vinyasa Yoga, we hold each pose for approximately five breaths, which comes to about fifteen to twenty seconds. If you are a beginner and feel you need to start off holding for only three breaths, then do that, eventually working your way up to five. Similarly, if you are a more advanced student and want to hold the poses longer, you can do that, too. Be intuitive as to whether you need to shorten or lengthen your holding time. Remember, you are holding the *pose*—not your breath!

Core Stabilization

In each pose, we engage an abdominal "lock," called *uddiyana*. Uddiyana is a gentle lifting of the pit of the abdomen toward the spine that stabilizes your core, protects and supports your lower back, and causes you to move and breathe from your center. It is the grounding force that enables the rest of your body to take on a feeling of weightlessness.

To engage your abdominal lock, contract your belly and lift it up toward your spine. As you draw the navel inward, the abdominal muscles follow, creating a hollowness under the rib cage and driving the breath into the upper torso and chest. Re-

member not to force the contraction—it is meant to be gentle but constant.

Meditation

There is a prison in India called Tikun, which is one of the largest and was once considered one of the most wretched and violent prisons in all of the world. About ten years ago, a new superintendent was brought in to reform the system. One of the first things she did was institute an awareness-based meditation program for the prisoners. The course was a very intensive ten days in which the students sat unmoving and in total silence for eleven hours each day. Before long, the behavior of the inmates who did the course started to change for the better. What seemed like a simple act of sitting ended up radically transforming the hearts and minds of these inmates, and as a result, the entire prison itself.

We have heard stories about the awesome power of meditation, yet so few people actually do it. The illusion is that one day you'll be ready for meditation, but in your heart, you're always ready. If you wait for your mind and ego to say, "Sure, let's try it!" you may be waiting a very long time, because your mind will never believe it can get quiet or still enough on its own. There will always be resistance at first, but the key is to do it anyway. If not now, when?

When we resist and struggle against our natural peace—when we react, get angry, hold resentments, and worry—we reject the source of light within. In meditation, we let those emotions arise without aiming them at an external target. As you see an emotion, feel it, and let it pass, a deep purification takes place. When you come into stillness, you can intimately know the truth, and the experience of that truth that sets you free. Great transformation happens in our moment-to-moment willingness to drop whatever story we are telling ourselves and open our fearful heart. Sitting and staying with the present moment takes some effort, but our commitment to growth and to seeking the truth can help us to overcome the greatest part of the difficulty.

There are a lot of different styles of meditation. I practice and teach a very simple awareness-based style, where the goal is not to tune out the world around you, but to wake up to it. In each of the six weeks, we will do the same basic meditation, which I will walk you through below. What differs each week will be the focus of the meditation and the length of time you will sit (you will begin with five minutes in the morning and five in the evening, working your way up to thirty minutes at the beginning and end of your day). When I say focus, I don't mean something you will concentrate on or contemplate. Instead, these are *intentions* that you want to let flow past your brain and impress themselves on the deeper soil of your psyche.

The Basic Technique

The basic focus of this technique is to stay present and aware of your body, your breath, and your surroundings. When thoughts arise, which they invariably will, we will just notice them and let them go, coming back to your awareness of your body, breath, and surroundings.

Begin by finding a comfortable place to sit with your legs crossed. It is best not to sit on your bed, because we're conditioned to see the bed as a place for sleeping. You may want to place a few cushions on the floor or fold up a few blankets to put underneath you. Or, you can sit upright in a straight-backed chair. Either way, arrange yourself so that your legs are slightly lower than your hips (this can help to keep your legs from falling asleep), maintaining an erect yet relaxed posture. Get comfortable, then get quiet and close your eyes.

Place your hands in your lap in a prayerlike position, fingertips touching and palms naturally coming apart. Breathe in and out, not manipulating the breath or trying to control it, just simply noticing as it flows in and out of your nostrils. Watch it rise and fall.

Bring your attention to your base. Feel your contact with the floor, chair, or whatever it is you are sitting on. Walk the fingers of your mind slowly up your spine, trailing your awareness upward, up through your head, until you come to your third eye center. Look through the center of your forehead with your eyes closed. You may see flashes of light or colors, or you may see nothing at all. Just watch this inner wall and notice whatever it is that you see.

Now bring your attention to your hands. Feel the energy flowing to your hands. Don't force your attention there; just feel and watch them with your mind's eye. Bring your attention to your thumbs, your first fingers, your second fingers, your third fingers, and your baby fingers. Shift your attention from one finger to another to center and anchor yourself. Bringing awareness to this fixed point on your anatomy bridges your mind and body; use your hands as an anchor to bring you back to the present moment if at any time you drift off during this meditation. Your hands are always there, always available to bring you right back into your breath and your body. Whenever your mind wanders, simply bring your attention back to your hands and begin again. That is your practice.

Now radiate your awareness into and throughout your whole body. Open your ears to the sounds around you, letting each one be a reference point to the present moment. Hearing grounds you in moment-to-moment awareness. Be perfectly present, perfectly relaxed. Do not manufacture any thoughts or stories about the sounds you hear. Simply let them flow in and out of your ears, holding on to nothing.

Begin to notice your thoughts. Step

HOW TO DEVELOP A DAILY MEDITATION PRACTICE

Meditation is a lifelong journey. Checking in daily with this profound practice impacts all areas of life and takes us way beyond feeling better into *being* better. The following are some suggestions in helping you establish your daily meditation habit:

- Meditate every morning before you do anything else, to center yourself for the day.
- Establish a distraction-free space for meditation.
- Decide how long you will sit before you begin to meditate, and set a clock or a timer to let you know when your time is finished.
- You can sit quietly, follow the described method below, or go to our website at www.baronbaptiste.com to attain one of the guided meditation CDs.
- Keep it pure and simple. Don't try to do anything or induce a certain state of mind; simply become more clear about what you are experiencing each moment.
- Stay in your body—it is an anchor to the present moment.

outside them and observe them, increasing the space between you and them. As you do this, notice that you are not your thoughts. They are separate from you, and you can let them go and still be present to observe your breath and root yourself to the present moment through your hands. Each time you notice you are thinking, release the thought and come back, again and again. As soon as you notice that you have gotten caught up in mental chatter or a story in your mind, you have freed yourself from it.

You may experience all kinds of sensations—for example, you may feel fidgety, uncomfortable, or itchy—but this is all just resistance. Just let the sensations go and begin again. If emotions rise to the surface, don't struggle to contain them. Let them come up and out for release. Feel your feelings without losing yourself in them.

Stay in this quiet and still space for as long as you have allotted for yourself. When you are ready, open your eyes.

The Most Commonly Asked Questions About Meditation

HOW CAN I STOP MY THOUGHTS?

The goal of meditation is not to stop our thinking or even clear our minds. In fact, that would be impossible. In the same way that our hearts beat, our minds think. Meditation is the practice of being less immersed in our thoughts and knowing the difference between thinking and being lost in thoughts. If we don't know the difference, we live in the stories in our heads and never come out of ourselves long enough to see the world as it really is.

Don't try to stop your thoughts. Don't block them: Let them come up, and then let them go. See your thoughts as clouds floating through the sky of your mind. Stand back and watch them drift by. This practice lets you see just how impermanent your thoughts really are, and takes away their power to rule your life. It teaches you the important truth that *you are not your thoughts.*

From time to time, you'll forget to be present and get wrapped up in your thoughts, but as often as you forget, remember to let them go and come back to your hands. Again and again, you simply begin again.

WHAT AM I SUPPOSED TO DO WITH ALL THE GREAT AND/OR CREATIVE IDEAS THAT COME UP WHILE I AM MEDITATING? AM I SUPPOSED TO JUST IGNORE THOSE AND GO ON MEDITATING?

That is exactly what you are supposed to do. This is a commitment question: Are you committed to your spiritual practice, or are you committed to it only as long as it is easy or convenient? If you made a sacred commitment to your spiritual path, it may be tempting to write down the profound thoughts when they come up, but the point is to let the thoughts go, no matter how juicy they are. The good news is that if your insights are really profound and really true to you, they will still be present for you when your meditation practice is done.

HOW DO I FIND THE TIME TO MEDITATE WHEN MY LIFE IS ALREADY SO BUSY?

No one ever says he doesn't have time to brush his teeth or take a shower, but people swear they can't find five minutes to be in stillness that will make them a better person. The bottom line is that you just need to make the commitment to setting aside a certain amount of time a day, and doing it. If you respect your commitment to it, you'll show up.

We can always find ways to carve out time if we really want to. When I am with my kids, they are always begging me to let them play on the computer, so I have them wait until my meditation time, and then I say, "Okay, you have thirty minutes." I set my egg timer and meditate in quiet for half an hour, because I know they won't be interrupting me. They are busy, I'm happy—it's a win-win situation.

HOW DO I KNOW IF I AM DOING IT RIGHT?

There is no right or wrong. There is just showing up and sitting with the

calmest determination you can find. It is important to give up the idea of being a "good" meditator or having any specific results. All that is required of you is just showing up, being present, and reaping the cumulative rewards. Sometimes the benefits are not immediately visible, but over time they will take effect. Over the years, you can look back and clearly see the subtle shifts in your mind, your perceptions—and your life.

WHAT DO I DO IF MY LEG FALLS ASLEEP?

That happens sometimes. You may go through all different kinds of sensations, from a tiny itch that starts to feel like torture to a tingling in your legs. I've had times when I've had pins and needles all over my entire body. The answer to what you should do is *nothing*. Do nothing. Continue to sit in committed stillness with strong determination and nonreactivity. Recognize this as just another bodily sensation and stay.

HOW DO I END MY PRACTICE?

The awareness-based style is all about presence and awareness, and if you are already present and aware, there is no ending that needs to happen to bring you back to your reality—you're already here. However, because you may have moments in which you drift off, you may want to wait until you have come back to your breath and the present moment, and then simply open your eyes.

WHAT DOES MEDITATION DO THAT YOGA DOES NOT?

Physical practice is great for your body and your nervous system, but meditation renews your mind and puts you in a better mental and spiritual space from which to move and flow. Meditation is the soul of your asana practice.

The Balancing Diet

Unlike a lot of other programs you may have read about or done, the diet section of this book is not a day-by-day regimen. It won't have menu plans or strict guidelines about what you should and should not eat. How can I speak of the need to be true to yourself and then presume to tell you how you should eat?

What I can provide you with is a framework that you can use to look within and approach your diet consciously, so that your common sense can guide what you eat. The more you come into your body, the more your bad habits will lose their hold on you and eventually give you up. It won't feel like a struggle; it will feel natural and right.

Having spent many years researching

different paths of nutrition, from cultures all over the world, I have found that the nutritional foundation of traditional Chinese medicine makes the most intuitive sense, because its entire premise is based on bringing the body back into balance. Disease, excess weight, and physical ailments arise because we are cluttered and out of balance. Like our minds, when our bodies are clear and balanced, we can receive the wisdom and vitality the winds of grace want to offer us. Then and only then do we lose weight and start to feel healthier and more alive.

Our American culture puts such emphasis on extremes when it comes to eating. We are either eating everything in sight or zero carbs. We are either too fat or too thin; we eat too much or too little. What we fail to realize, however, is that at all times we are in a cycle. We have different needs at different times, both throughout the year and in our own internal seasons. The goal is not to richochet from one extreme to another, but to artfully intuit where we are in the cycles at any given time, and to nourish our body accordingly so that we can move into a more healthful state of equilibrium and illumination.

In each week, you will be given a new insight into eating for balance. Beginning in Week One, which is all about awakening, you will learn how to consciously identify your particular body pattern, so you can know what foods will help bring your personal ecosystem back into balance. The theme of Week Two is vitality, and we will talk about the extraordinary value of replacing empty, soulless foods with fresh, life-giving ones. In Week Three, the week of equanimity, we will focus on cravings and how to handle those powerful internal storms when they blow through. Week Four is the three-day fruit fast, which will wholly cleanse your system so that you can energetically feel the theme of the week, which is receiving the radiance. Week Five is about centering, and immediately following the cleanse, we will talk about how we can re-ground our bodies through intake of essential minerals. Finally, we come to Week Six, the week of triumph. Here we will have a chance to review the effects the past five weeks of new habits have had on us, and consciously choose which we want to incorporate into our daily lives going forward.

The entire purpose of the balancing diet is to bring you back into your natural state. If you need to lose weight, that is what will happen. Chances are that any physical ailments that have plagued you will start to disappear once you bring your body's ecosystem into balance. All that is not naturally of you will drop away; all the excess weight, lethargy, and whatever else holds you back will disappear as you come to your state of healthful equilibrium.

The Excavation Questions

The excavation questions for each week are not meant to send you off on some psychological head trip of why you do this or that. That is the intellectual path of questioning that only leads you further into your head and away from your heart. These questions are meant to just bring to your awareness the beliefs, ideas, and scenarios in your life that are holding you back. There is nothing for you to figure out and nothing for you to do with the answers that arise other than simply to become conscious of and clarify them so that you can ultimately let them go. Ask any recovering addict and he or she will tell you that the first step of any recovery process is awareness. The whole purpose of this journey is to overthrow the regime that is currently running your life, and with that must come a letting go.

I recommend that you set some time aside each week to write out your responses to these questions. I often find—as have many of my students—that the way I think I might answer a question in the abstract looks very different when I start to commit my response to paper. There is something very revealing and cathartic about the process of writing, as it forces us to express ourselves in a slower, more deliberate way. Also, it helps to have your responses recorded, because as time goes by, it can be easy to forget the insight that seemed so profound only a few days ago.

The Seventh Day

As the Bible says, there is a time for work and a time for rest. The seventh day of each week will be a day of active rest, for you to let go, let loose, and enjoy yourself and your life. It is important to do this while undergoing the upheaval of transformation so that you can assimilate and absorb all you have done, while at the same time replenishing your energies.

In our crazy world, we don't encourage real rest. We have to make the space for it. In the West, we never really take rest—we watch TV (which is a stimulant) or go out to dinner, to the movies, or sporting events. But is that truly rest?

True rest involves some time in isolation, when you close your sense doors and regenerate. Don't rush to fill the space and silence with sounds and people. When you work, work hard, but when you rest, remember to rest fully and completely.

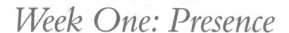

Week One: Presence

SOMEONE ONCE ASKED THE BUDDHA, "ARE YOU A GOD?"

"NO," HE REPLIED.

"Are you a saint?"

"No."

"Then what are you?" they asked.

"Awake."

How many of us are really awake? It is so easy for us to get swept up in the emotional white sugar of the world: confusion, reactivity, fear, demands of work, parenting, money. When we feel crazy or out of control at any point in our lives, it is because we have left our bodies and lost contact with our essential selves. Our culture leads us to believe that our problem is with food, or our boss, or our relationships, but really, these things are not the problem.

The problem is that we have disconnected from consciousness and gone to sleep.

Growing up, I often felt like my parents were too busy. I resented them for not slowing down enough to just spend time hanging out with me. Now, as an adult, I see how seductive the world can be and how easy it is to get carried away by blind ambition and constant doing, which in the end leads to a life that is less fulfilled, if not one full of regrets.

As a parent of three boys of my own, I've made a contract with my kids that a certain amount of time I devote to work, but the rest of the time I will keep my focus with them. That means full presence, seeing everything else as a diversion or distraction. Physically hanging up the phone or turning off the computer is one thing, but emptying my mind enough to be completely with them is another. It is so easy to be somewhere and not really *be there*. I've taught them to call me on it when I'm not being present with them. "Dad, you're not really here," they'll shout at me, and it reminds me that every moment I spend with them is irreplaceable, precious, and sacred. I get only one chance with them. So I'll turn off the phone, the e-mail, and the general micromanaging of my life and just be with them. My ego screams out that there is so much to do, but I've learned that staying present in anything is a practice. As often as I forget and get distracted, I must remember and simply begin again.

If at any point you realize that you have disconnected, you can take a time-out, come back, and wake up. You can reconnect to your higher power—the Tao, which is the law that creates and permeates the whole of existence. We live so much of our lives at an outward level, but here is a chance to consciously go inward. In Week One, your focus is on waking up and becoming fully present to your body, mind, and life. Most important, though, begin to see the underlying factors that are contributing to wherever you feel stuck in your life. When we act out compulsively and lack self-control, we say, "How can I

be so weak? Why don't I have any willpower?" But the truth is that our addictive, acting-out behavior does not represent a lack of power. In fact, it takes a lot of power to systematically sabotage every day of your life.

Feeling controlled by our problems, behaviors, and addictions is not an issue of powerlessness. The issue is that we are turning our power against ourselves. What many of us need to do is to wake up and heal the underlying relationship to ourselves. Wisdom does not focus on the form that our dysfunction takes: the overeating, self-sabotaging, dramatizing, or whatever other self-destructive behaviors we engage in. Instead, we need to get present to what is under there—what these behaviors are masking.

The line from the Bible that I quoted in Law 1: Seek the Truth says that when you know the truth, the truth will set you free. What is there to be set free from? For many of us, it is our own delusions and problems. When we awaken to the truth that is causing these problems, we are set free from our slavery to food, alcohol, overeating, obsessive thinking, or whatever binds us and weighs us down. As we wake up, we become more compassionate with ourselves. As we gain new insights about our thoughts and behaviors, we recognize that we are not hopelessly defective or demented. We realize that struggling and fighting with our symptoms only entangles us more deeply, and using willpower to change a habit is like trying to think away a broken leg. We don't heal deep wounds with surface Band-Aids. If we are truly and permanently to be set free, we need to get quiet enough to see the underlying truth of our behaviors and self-defeating patterns.

For all four parts of your practice this week, your focus will be on awakening. The first week's yoga practice, which is twenty minutes long, will start to bring you into your body and your breath. For some of you, the first week will be all about burning off the stuff and stress of life so that you can get to the point where you can really exhale. The focus of your meditation practice will be to cultivate full awareness of the present moment. In the first week of the Balancing Diet, you will bring awareness to your particular body pattern and learn how you can best start to nourish yourself accordingly. Lastly, the excavation questions will shine a light on the dark corners of your mind, where we all store the beliefs and patterns that are holding us back in life.

Week One Yoga Practice
20 Minutes

AS WITH ALL THE SEQUENCES IN *40 DAYS TO PERSONAL REVOLUTION*, THE TWENTY-MINUTE PRACTICE BEGINS WITH THE FOLLOWING THREE INTEGRATION POSES:

Child's Pose, Downward Facing Dog, and Ragdoll. These poses allow us to come into our bodies and shift our minds from distraction to direction.

Pose 1: Child's Pose

Child's Pose awakens the connection between your breath and your body. It is a resting pose that can also be used at any time during your practice, whenever you feel you need it.

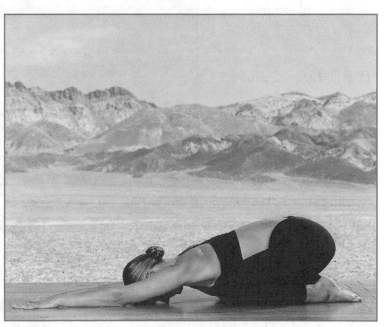

Pose 1: Child's Pose

Building Blocks

1. From a standing position, come to your hands and knees.
2. Point your toes so the tops of your feet are flat on the mat.
3. Keep your big toes together and widen your knees to the outer edges of your mat.
4. Shift the weight of your hips back so your butt rests on your heels.
5. Extend your arms straight out in front of you, palms facing down.
6. Bring your forehead to the floor, close your eyes, and just rest.

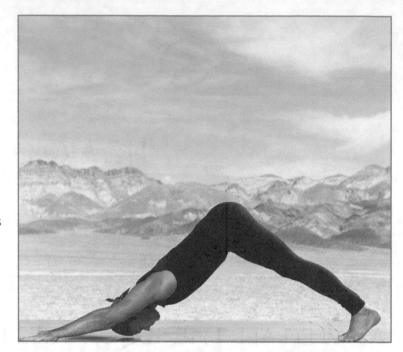

Pose 2: Downward Facing Dog (Adho Mukha Svanasana)

Pose 2: Downward Facing Dog (Adho Mukha Svanasana)

Downward Facing Dog engages your whole being: it calms your nervous system, engages an overall flexible strength, decompresses your spine, tones and strengthens your arms, opens the arches of your feet, sculpts and lengthens

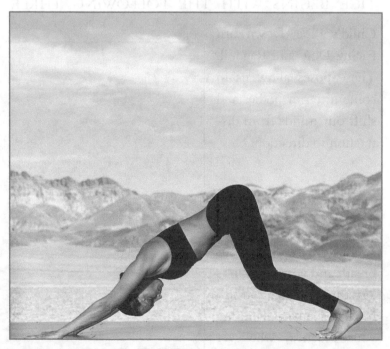

Downward Facing Dog (Adho Mukha Svanasana), modification

your thighs, and is an amazing shoulder opener. It can be an active home base for you during your practice, as it is both dynamic and restful at the same time.

The first Downward Dog of the practice is about checking in with your body. Where are you as you begin this practice? Where is your mind? Drop your day and come into your body.

Building Blocks

1. From Child's Pose, stretch your arms out in front of you, palms on the floor, hands shoulder width apart.
2. Curl your toes under and press your tail high, straightening your legs.
3. Walk your feet toward the back of your mat and your hands forward to create a nice, long base.
4. Tilt your tailbone up and create length in your spine. From the side you should look like an inverted V.
5. Roll your shoulder blades down your back, spreading them apart, rotating your arms so the pits of your elbows face each other.
6. Press down into the triads of your hands: the knuckles of your thumb and index finger and the space in between.
7. Rest your eyes on one spot. Breathe deeply and freely, letting the layers of tension fall away.

Alignment

- Press your palms flat, fingers evenly spread apart.
- Press your thighbones back toward the wall behind you.
- Contract and activate your quadriceps.
- Pull your hips back and tilt your tailbone up.
- Pull your navel toward your spine for upward lift.
- Drop the shoulder blades down your back, bringing the elbows in toward each other.
- Drop your head and rest your eyes on one point.

One of the most common complaints beginning yoga students have is that their wrists hurt. If Downward Facing Dog causes strain on your wrists, put more emphasis to pressing down through the knuckles of your index fingers. This will help to properly distribute your weight and stabilize your wrists.

Also, remember to rotate your shoulders down your back. Imagine you have two pickle jars, one beneath each palm: open the right one in a clockwise direction and the left one counterclockwise, to get a sense of this motion.

Finally, use your whole body force to lift up and out of your wrists. Press your thigh bones back and lift your tailbone to the sky, so as to not jam all your body weight into your wrist joints.

Pose 3: Ragdoll

Ragdoll releases the back of your body and continues to awaken your biochemistry. Like Downward Facing Dog, it has an inversion element to it, which revitalizes the nervous system and helps to create hormonal harmony.

Building Blocks

1. From Downward Facing Dog, walk your feet up to your hands. Feet are hip width apart and parallel.
2. Bring hands to opposite biceps.
3. Let your weight roll into the balls of your feet.
4. Drop your head and let your neck hang, soft and free. Shake your head yes and no a few times, to make sure you are really letting go.
5. Soften your eyes and set them on a point behind you.
6. Hang down and *breathe*.

Alignment

- Press the soles of your feet into your mat.
- Bend your knees slightly to protect them and your lower back.
- Sway your hips forward so they are over your heels.
- Keep your legs active and strong, the upper body relaxed and free.
- Press your sitting bones up toward the sky.
- Let your head hang, creating length through your neck.

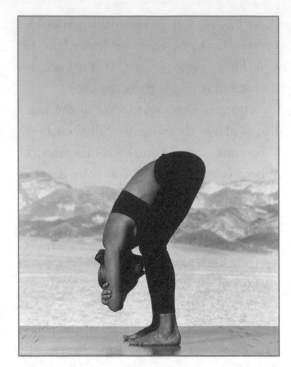

Pose 3: Ragdoll

Modification

Bend your knees as much as you need to if you feel any tightness in your lower back.

Sun Salutation A

Following the integration poses, we move into Sun Salutation A and Sun Salutation B. In Baptiste Power Vinyasa Yoga, Sun Salutation A is also used as a connecting link between poses in order to keep the flow, or vinyasa moving. It is like the palate cleanser in between courses. Wherever I say to "go through the vinyasa or vinyasa A," I am referring to Sun Salutation A.

Pose 4: Samasthiti

Samasthiti means "standing at attention" in Sanskrit. It cultivates body awareness and helps establish your personal stature from the onset of your practice.

Building Blocks

1. From Ragdoll, toe/heel your feet together so the big toes are touching.
2. With soft knees, roll up to standing one vertebra at time.
3. Stand up straight at the front of your mat.
4. Drive your legs down into the earth and lift your sternum up toward the heavens, creating traction between the soles of your feet and the top of your head.
5. Pull the tops of your shoulders back and relax them, hands hanging by your sides.
6. Gaze forward and stand tall with a natural integrity.

Alignment

- Root your feet to the earth and lift your arches.
- Press the inner edges of your feet together.
- Center your hips and scoop the front of your pelvis up as though you were holding a cup of water in your pelvic bowl.
- Open your chest and lift your sternum as you soften the front ribs.
- Pull the tops of your shoulders back and down, away from your ears.

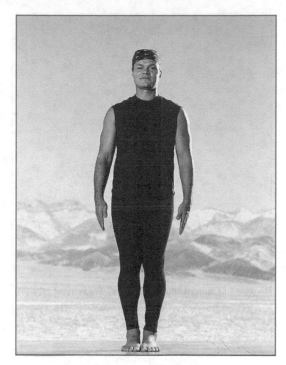

Pose 4: Samasthiti

- Engage your hands and activate your fingertips.

Pose 5: Mountain Pose (Tadasana)

This pose reverses and relieves the constant gravitational stress on the body, lengthening and creating openness in the front of the torso, neck, chest, and shoulders.

Building Blocks

1. From Samasthiti, spin your palms outward.
2. Inhale, lift your chin slightly, and sweep your hands up sideways, stopping when they are shoulder width apart above your head.

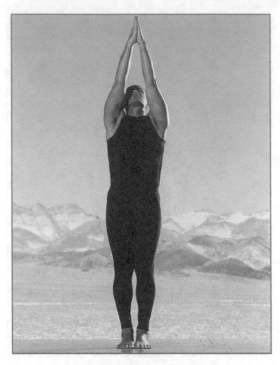

Pose 5: Mountain Pose (Tadasana)

3. Gaze at a point directly above you on the ceiling.

Alignment

Same as for Samasthiti, plus:

- Reach your fingertips to the sky and root your feet down into the earth, creating length and space in your entire body.
- Eyes rest up on the ceiling on one point.
- Pull your belly in toward your spine.

Pose 6: Standing Forward Bend (Uttanasana)

This forward bend stretches the lower back and hamstrings. As with all inversions, it also harmonizes the brain chemistry.

Building Blocks

1. From Mountain Pose, exhale and swan-dive forward with a straight spine, hinging at your hips.
2. Sweep your arms down sideways, bringing your fingers to the floor on either side of your toes.
3. Press your chest down into your legs.
4. Let your head hang down with your neck free.

Alignment

- Keep your feet active.
- Stack your shins, knees, thighbones, and hips in a vertical line.

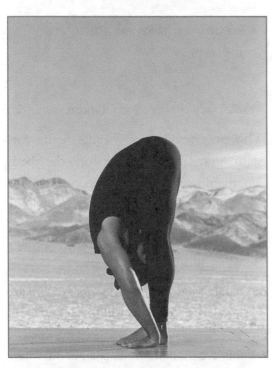

Pose 6: Standing Forward Bend (Uttanasana)

- Spread your sitting bones away from each other.
- Focus on drawing the crown of your head down toward the mat, using your hands around your ankles as leverage.
- Breathe into whatever tightness you may feel in your hamstrings or lower back.
- Allow your eyes to stay soft.

Modification

If this strains your lower back, bend your knees.

Pose 7: Halfway Lift (Urdhva Mukha Uttanasana)

The Halfway Lift continues to stretch the hamstrings and lower back, and also elongates the spine and tones the abdominal obliques.

Building Blocks

1. From Standing Forward Bend, keep your feet together and place your fingertips on the floor to the outer edges of your feet, in line with your toes.
2. Inhale as you lift your torso halfway up to a flat back.
3. Gaze at a spot on the floor six inches ahead of your toes.

Alignment

- Place your fingertips on the floor in line with your toes.

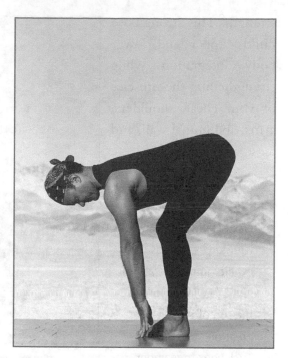

Pose 7: Halfway Lift
(Urdhva Mukha Uttanasana), modification

- Press your tall back and your chest forward.
- Extend and lengthen your spine.
- Drop your shoulder blades down your back and away from your ears.
- Bring your chin toward your chest so your neck is in line with your entire spine.

Modification

Bend your knees as much as you need to in order to maintain a flat back. Place your hands on your shins.

Pose 8: High Push-Up (Dandasana)

Dandasana literally translates to "staff," which is a symbol of great power and strength. This strong pose builds upper and lower body integration while strengthening the muscles of your chest, shoulders, arms, abdominal wall, and legs.

Building Blocks

1. From Halfway Lift, bend your knees, and as you exhale, jump or walk your feet back so you are at the top of a push-up position.
2. Tuck your toes under, standing on the balls of your feet.
3. Stack your shoulders over your wrists.
4. Engage your quadriceps.
5. Lift your belly to your spine.
6. Set your gaze at a spot on the mat between your hands.

Alignment

- Engage your quads and lift the front of your thighs, simultaneously pressing back through your heels.

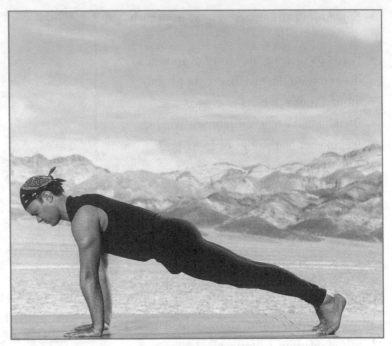

Pose 8: High Push-Up (Dandasana)

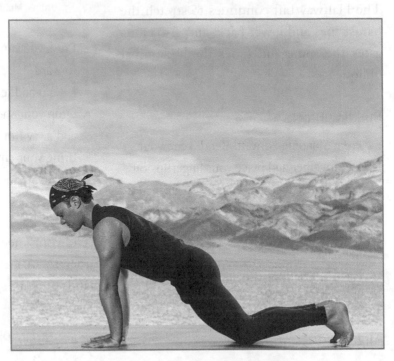

High Push-Up (Dandasana), modification

Your breath is key for maintaining your fluidity in the vinyasa. It is like the lubricating motor oil for the engine of a car.

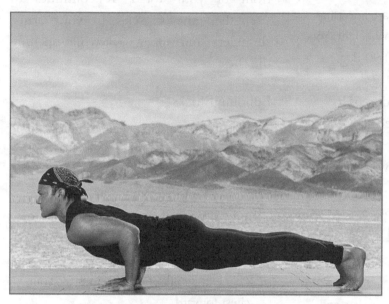
Pose 9: Low Push-Up (Chaturanga Dandasana)

- Stack your shoulder joints, elbows, and wrists all in one line.
- Use your core power and your legs to help you hold this pose.
- Gently lift and contract your abdomen.

Modification

Drop your knees to the mat to lessen the intensity of this pose.

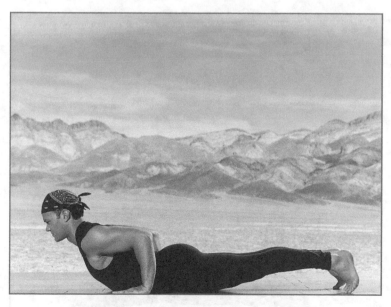
Low Push-Up (Chaturanga Dandasana), modification

Pose 9: Low Push-Up (Chaturanga Dandasana)

Chaturanga encourages full-body stabilization and coordinated force of your entire musculature. This can be a challenging pose for newer students, but remember that we must step out of our comfort zone if we want to transform.

Building Blocks

1. From High Push-Up, exhale and bend your elbows.
2. Move your upper body forward as you lower your torso until you are hovering with your shoulders at elbow height. Your elbows should form perfect 90-degree angles.
3. Engage your belly and quadriceps to distribute the burden of weight evenly.
4. As in High Push-Up, tuck your tailbone down toward your heels.
5. Keep your chin slightly raised.
6. Gaze forward and breathe!

Alignment

- Stack your elbows over your wrists and tuck them into your ribs.
- Shoulders hover at elbow level.
- Balance on the balls of your feet.
- Engage and lift your quadriceps and belly.
- Slide your shoulder blades down the back.

Modification

As in High Push-Up, you can drop your knees. If you need further modification, drop your chest down to the mat as well.

Pose 10: Upward Facing Dog (Urdhva Mukha Svanasana)

Upward Facing Dog stretches the entire front of your torso. It continues to strengthen the muscles in your arms, shoulders, and upper back while opening the chest.

Building Blocks

1. From Low Push-Up, inhale and press down on your hands, scooping your chest and belly up.
2. Move your torso forward and through your arms as you roll over the tops of your toes, the tops of your feet pressing into your mat.
3. Pull your shoulders back and press your chest forward.

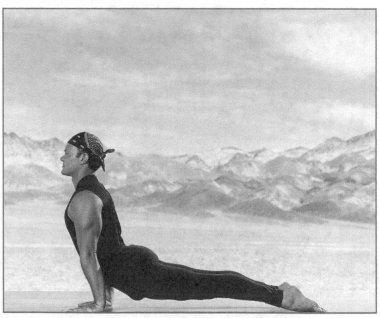

Pose 10: Upward Facing Dog (Urdhva Mukha Svanasana)

4. Drive down through your arms and the tops of your feet; engage your legs.
5. Gaze forward.

Alignment

- Press your palms and the tops of your feet down into your mat.
- Engage your quadriceps, glutes, and abdomen to lift the front of your thighs off the mat.
- Spin your inner thighs up, keeping your toes on the floor.
- Stack your shoulders, elbows, and wrists in one vertical line.
- Draw your shoulders back, away from your ears.
- Keep your neck in a neutral line with your spine.

Modification

If you feel this in your lower back, bend your arms, tuck your elbows into your sides, and rest your belly on the floor.

Repeat Pose 2: Downward Facing Dog (Adho Mukha Svanasana)

The building blocks and alignment for Downward Facing Dog are the same as when you did this pose earlier. To move into Downward Facing Dog from Upward Facing Dog, exhale, and in one fluid motion drive the back of your thighs to the wall behind you until you are in an inverted V. Adjust your hands and feet as necessary to come into proper alignment.

In Sun Salutations, hold Downward Facing Dog for five full breaths.

Pose 11: Jump Forward

The Jump Forward links one pose to another and helps to build heat.

Building Blocks

1. On the fifth exhalation of Downward Facing Dog, empty your lungs completely and press your thighs back even further.
2. Pull your belly up to your spine.
3. Look at your hands, bend your knees, and, using your abdominal stability and upper body force, jump your feet forward between your hands.

Modification

You can walk your feet forward one at a time until you are more comfortable with the Jump Forward.

Don't use momentum here. Use your upper body force and your abdominal muscles to float forward. You want to be light and easy, landing softly without a sound. Remember, Buddha said, "Make yourself light."

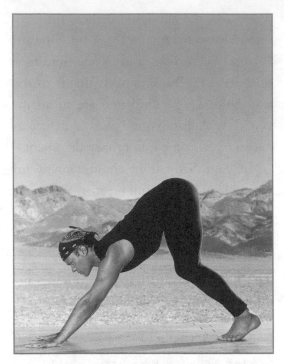

Pose 11: Jump Forward, starting position

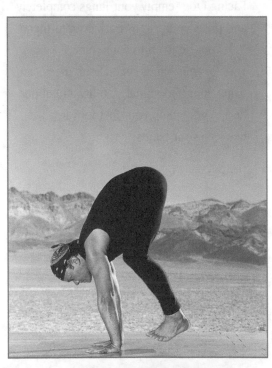

Jump Forward, finishing position

To finish the Sun Salutation A, after you jump or walk forward, come into Halfway Lift (Pose 7), then fold forward into Standing Forward Bend (Pose 6). From there, sweep your arms up sideways until you are standing in Mountain Pose (Pose 5). Make sure to engage your abdominal lock as you come up. Then drop your arms and come back to Samasthiti (Pose 4). Repeat Sun Salutation A two times, then proceed to Sun Salutation B.

Sun Salutation B

Sun Salutation B continues to build the internal heat. Much of this vinyasa is the same as Sun Salutation A, with a few new poses included.

Pose 12: Thunderbolt (Utkatasana)

Utkatasana translates to "powerful," much like a thunderbolt. This is a very dynamic pose that increases the heart rate and stimulates the circulatory and metabolic systems.

Building Blocks

1. From Samasthiti, inhale as you bend your knees deeply to 90 degrees and bring your arms up alongside your ears. Arms are shoulder width apart, palms facing each other.
2. Squat down as if you were sitting in a chair, bringing your hips and tail slightly back.

3. Dip your hips low and press your heart high.
4. Spread your shoulder blades apart.
5. Pull your fingers skyward, up out of their knuckles.
6. Spin your pinky fingers in toward each other, rotating your thumbs outward.
7. Gently lift your chin and look up through your hands.
8. Hold for five breaths.

Alignment

- Lift your toes and shift the majority of your body weight into your heels.
- Keep your hips/tail slightly back.
- Drop your hips and lift your heart and hands.
- Spin your arms so your little fingers move in and your thumbs move outward.
- Spread your scapula to broaden your upper back.

Connecting Vinyasa

After the fifth breath of Thunderbolt, lower your hips two more inches for an additional breath, then exhale and hinge forward. Wait until your hands reach the mat or your ankles, whichever you can reach, then straighten your legs, coming into Standing Forward Bend (6). Go

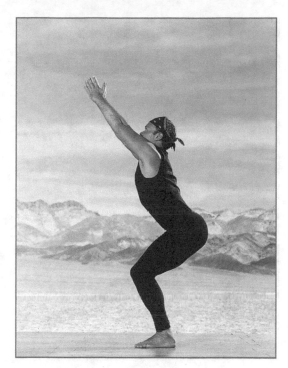

Pose 12: Thunderbolt (Utkatasana)

through steps 7 through 10 of Sun Salutation A (Halfway Lift, High Push-Up, Low Push-Up, Upward Facing Dog) and end in Downward Facing Dog (2).

Pose 13: Warrior I (Virabhadrasana I)

Warrior I is a dynamic pose. It creates a powerful integration of leg strength and fluid flexibility of the hips, and also prepares the body for backbends later in the practice.

Remember, if you are not relaxing, you are reacting. Can you relax with what is, even if it is hard? Can you meet the stress of a challenging pose with grace rather than resistance?

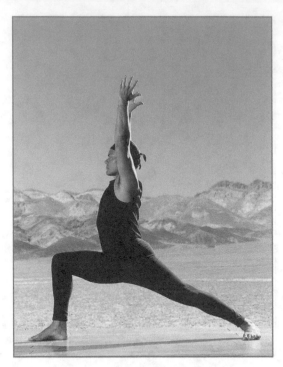

Pose 13: Warrior I (Virabhadrasana I)

Building Blocks

1. From Downward Facing Dog, exhale and lunge your right foot forward to your right hand, bending your front knee to 90 degrees.
2. Spin your back foot flat to a 60-degree angle, with your heels on one line.
3. On the in breath, sweep your hands up over your head on either side of your ears (like in Thunderbolt).
4. Face your palms toward each other with the little fingers spinning in and the thumbs spinning out.

5. Take powerful aim and fuse your eyes to one point.

Alignment

- Keep your heels on one line.
- Lift the inner ankle of the back foot and press into its outer edge.
- Dip your front leg down to 90 degrees so the thigh and shin form a right angle.
- Square your hips, pulling your right hip back and your left hip forward.
- Scoop your tailbone down and forward.
- Rotate both thighbones in a clockwise direction.
- Reach your heart and arms skyward.

Connecting Vinyasa

From Warrior I, place your hands on your mat on either side of your front foot and step back into High Push-Up Position (8). Go through Vinyasa A (High Push-Up, Low Push-Up, Upward Facing Dog, Downward Facing Dog). From Downward Facing Dog, step your left foot forward and spin your right foot flat into Warrior I, following all the same instructions as above, except in reverse.

Go through Vinyasa A again (High Push-Up, Low Push-Up, Upward Facing Dog, Downward Facing Dog). Take five deep breaths in Downward Dog. On the

You should be able to balance an orange on the top of your front thigh in this pose. If necessary, dip down lower to get your front thigh parallel to the floor.

last breath, exhale completely and Jump Forward (11). With your feet firmly on the mat, bend your knees and sweep back up again into Thunderbolt (12). Hold Thunderbolt for another five breaths, then fold forward into Standing Forward Bend (6) and begin another Sun Salutation B from there.

Repeat Sun Salutation B two full times, then go through the steps of Sun Salutation B until you are in Warrior I, right foot forward. This time, hold Warrior I for five full breaths.

Pose 14: Warrior II
(Virabhadrasana II)

Warrior II is an excellent hip-opening pose that sculpts the muscles of the buttocks and thighs. Beyond the physical, it hones your power of concentration. Through your focused gaze, it teaches you how to streamline your power, energetically bringing your mind from distraction to direction.

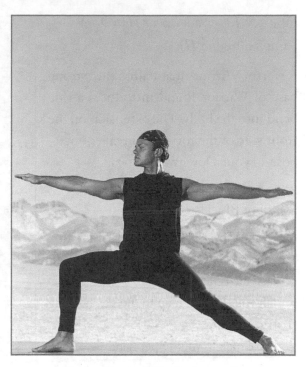

Pose 14: Warrior II (Virabhadrasana II)

Building Blocks

1. From Warrior I, square your hips and chest to the side wall and open your arms out to the sides at shoulder height, so they are over your thighs, palms facing down.
2. Gaze strongly and steadily at the middle fingernail of your right hand.
3. Hold for five breaths.

Alignment

- Press through the outer edge of your back foot.
- Stretch the mat apart with your feet.
- Stack the front knee over the ankle in a vertical line.
- Dip your hips down so your front thigh is parallel to the floor.
- Rotate your inner thighs out and away from each other.
- Lift your belly, spine, and chest.
- Stack your shoulders over your hips.
- Drop your shoulder blades down your back.
- Reach through both arms and fingertips as if you were being pulled apart.

Pose 15: Reverse Warrior (Parivrtta Virabhadrasana II)

Reverse Warrior maintains the strong base of Warrior II and introduces a side bend into the body. The extension on the front side of the torso is a great counter-pose to your Downward Dogs.

Building Blocks

1. From Warrior II, drop your back arm to your back leg, spin your front palm up to face the ceiling.
2. Lift your front arm up to the sky, bending back slightly.
3. Gaze high to your upper hand.

Alignment

Same as for Warrior II, plus roll the left knee out toward the left toe.

Connecting Vinyasa

Exhale and bring your front arm back to Warrior II. Helicopter your arms down and step back into High Push-Up. Go through the vinyasa (High to Low Push-Up, Upward Facing Dog, Downward Facing Dog). Step your left foot forward into Warrior I, and repeat the sequence of Warrior I, Warrior II, and Reverse Warrior on the left side. After the fifth breath in Reverse Warrior, go through the vinyasa again, ending in Downward Facing Dog. From Downward Facing Dog, drop your

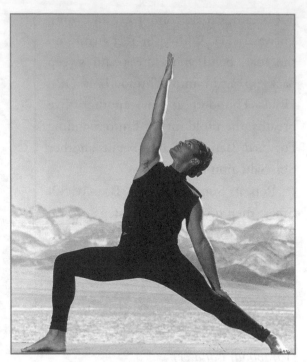

Pose 15: Reverse Warrior (Parivrtta Virabhadrasana II)

knees to the floor, lift your feet, cross your ankles, and roll over your feet to your seat in preparation for the next pose, Boat Pose.

Pose 16: Boat Pose (Navasana)

Navasana is a core-strengthening pose that creates whole-body integration and balance. Abdominal work is key to any healthy yoga practice, because strong abdominals take unnecessary pressure off your lower back. Building core muscles creates an inner strength and stability that gives you a deeper seat of power and balance throughout your body.

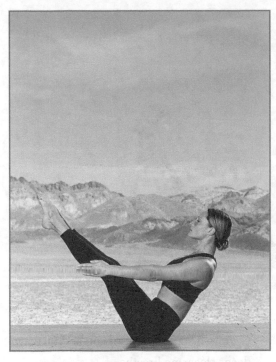

Pose 16: Boat Pose (Navasana)

Building Blocks

1. From the seated position, extend your legs straight to a 45-degree angle as you reach your arms forward, parallel to the floor.
2. Contract your abdominal wall and lift your sternum.
3. Gaze forward and breathe.

Alignment

- Balance on your tail and sitting bones.
- Use your core power to raise your legs and torso.
- Keep your lower back as straight as possible (avoid rounding or overarching).
- Press your inner thighs together.
- Activate your feet.
- Draw your sternum up to the sky.
- Reach your arms forward and activate your hands.

Modification

You can either bend your knees slightly or work with one foot on the floor if lifting both legs feels too strenuous. You can also keep your hands on the floor as you extend your legs straight to maintain balance.

Connecting Vinyasa

After the fifth breath, bend your knees and cross your feet in front of you. Place your hands down on the mat in front of your knees, roll forward, and lift your whole body off the floor for one breath. Come down and repeat the sequence of Navasana

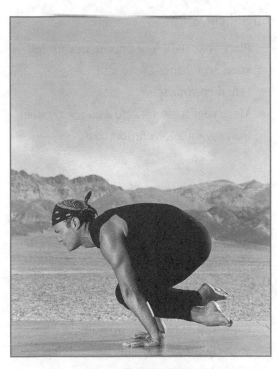

Boat Pose (Navasana), step 2

and the cross-and-lift four times, ending in the seated position with the soles of your feet on the floor and your knees bent.

Pose 17: Seated Half Pigeon (Urdhva Mukha Sukhasana)

Seated Half Pigeon is a hip-opening pose that releases the periformis muscles, which can get very tight in athletes and those who sit in a chair all day.

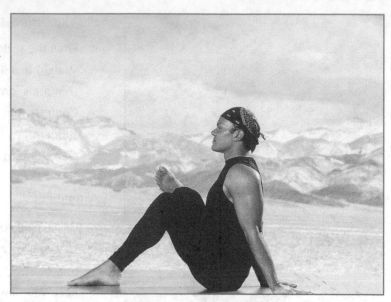

Pose 17: Seated Half Pigeon (Urdhva Mukha Sukhasana)

We store a lot of emotional tension in our hips, so at times these poses can feel pretty intense. I like to call the sensations that come up the "pains of purification." The key is to remember to breathe way down deep into any tightness or resistance you feel. Once you open your hips, your whole body begins to come into a more fluid alignment.

Building Blocks

1. From the seated position after Navasana, place your hands on the floor about eight inches behind you, palms down, fingers facing the back wall.
2. Cross your right foot over the top of your left thigh. Your shin is parallel to the floor.
3. Use your hands to walk your torso forward and press your chest toward your legs.

4. Gaze to a spot in front of you and take five deep, cleansing breaths.

Alignment

- Place your right foot outside of your left knee, so it hangs in the air.
- Lengthen your spine.
- Move your torso forward as a lever, rather than caving into your low back.

Pose 18: Three-Legged Tabletop (Arda Purvottanasana)

Three-Legged Tabletop is an excellent counterpose for hip work.

Building Blocks

1. From Seated Half Pigeon, walk your hands back eight inches, palms flat and fingers facing forward.

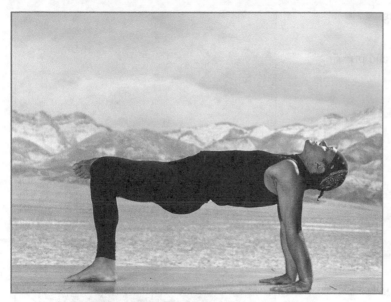

Pose 18: Three-Legged Tabletop (Arda Purvottanasana)

Modification

If it hurts your neck to drop your head back, simply bring your chin up toward your chest.

Connecting Vinyasa

After five breaths, bring your chin back into your chest and lower your hips down. Straighten your legs out in front of you in preparation for the next pose, the Staff.

2. With your leg still crossed, inhale and press down through your arms, hands, and lower foot, straightening your elbows and lifting your hips up high.
3. Drop your head so the crown of your head is facing the floor.
4. Gaze to the back wall.

Alignment

- Press your palms and your lower foot down into the floor.
- Stack your shoulders over your wrists.
- Move your shoulder blades in toward each other.
- Press down through your hands and foot to lift your hips higher.

Pose 19: The Staff (Dandasana)

This pose strengthens and awakens the whole body, toning the legs while releasing the spine and hips.

Building Blocks

1. Sit on the mat with your legs straight, strong, and active.
2. Bring your hands alongside your hips, palms down.
3. Press your thighs toward the floor.
4. Lift your chest and press your palms down into the earth.
5. Gently suck your sacrum and abdomen inward.

Alignment

- Press the inner edges of your feet forward.
- Activate your toes.

- Maintain straight, strong legs.
- Keep your spine straight.
- Continue lifting your chest and pressing your palms down.

Pose 20: Single-Legged Boat (Ekapadanavasana)

This pose stabilizes your core and helps develop postural stature.

Building Blocks

1. From the Staff, bend your right leg and place your right foot flat on the mat.
2. Bend the extended left leg, taking hold of the foot or calf with both hands.
3. Straighten the leg upward directly in front of you.
4. Let go of the leg and bring both arms parallel to the floor, as in regular Boat Pose.

Alignment

- Lift your sacrum.
- Lift your spine.
- Relax your shoulders.
- Fully engage your lifted leg.
- Radiate through your upper foot and toes.

Connecting Vinyasa

After five breaths, lower your leg and arms. Bend your left knee, same as the right, so the left foot is also flat on the mat, in preparation for the next pose.

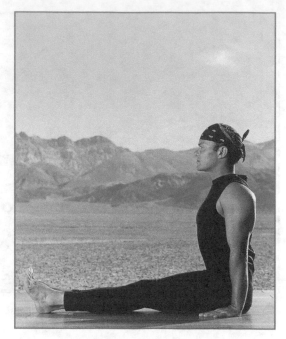

Pose 19: The Staff (Dandasana)

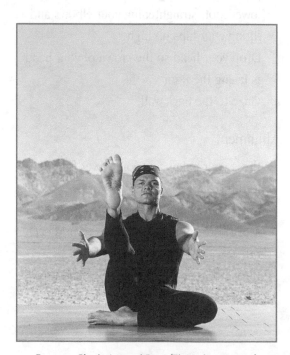

Pose 20: Single-Legged Boat (Ekapadanavasana)

Pose 21: Lifted Leg Pose (Crunchasana)

This pose is a deep stretch for the legs. It integrates the upper and lower body, develops core strength (teaching the abdominal lock), and develops spinal integrity and overall structural awareness.

Building Blocks

1. Sitting on both buttocks with your knees bent, tuck the left foot underneath the right buttock and drop the right knee to the floor.
2. Take the right foot with both hands (or behind the knee—wherever you can reach and still maintain a straight spine).
3. Holding the foot (or behind the knee), lift your leg and straighten it as much as you can.
4. Lift your chest and spine.
5. Emphasize your abdominal lock.
6. Relax your neck.
7. Gaze forward.

Alignment

- Continually lift your chest and spine. It is more important to have a straight spine than a straight leg.
- Keep your abdominal lock engaged.

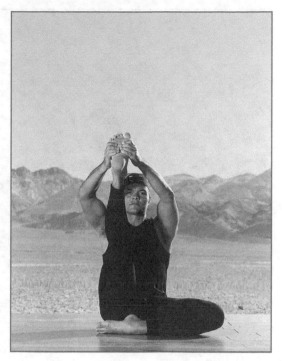

Pose 21: Lifted Leg Pose (Crunchasana)

- Maintain a deep and rhythmic ujjayi breath.

Pose 22: Twisting Lifted Leg Pose (Parivrtta Crunchasana)

This pose offers all the same benefits as Lifted Leg Pose, plus it adds a twisting movement that rinses out the internal organs.

This is a strong stretch for most people, so do not force it or be aggressive. Just apply effort and wait for the musculature to release.

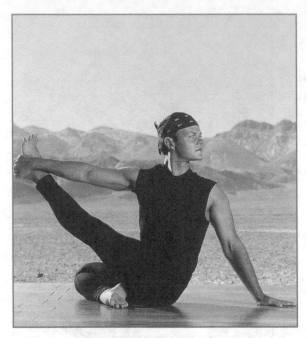

Pose 22: Twisting Lifted Leg Pose (Parivritta Crunchasana)

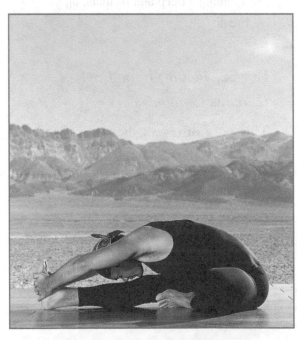

Pose 23: Easy Forward Bend (Janu Sirsasana)

Building Blocks

1. From Lifted Leg Pose, bring the upper leg across the center line of your body.
2. Release your left hand (the hand is opposite the lifted leg) and bring your left arm behind you, placing the palm flat on the floor.
3. Lift your chest and spine and twist to the left, using your back arm as leverage.
4. Relax your neck.
5. Gaze over your left shoulder.

Alignment

- On the in breath, lift your chest and spine. On the out breath, work the rotation of your torso.
- Emphasize your abdominal lock.
- Maintain a deep, rhythmic breath.

Connecting Vinyasa

After five breaths, release the lifted leg and bring your torso back to center.

Pose 23: Easy Forward Bend (Janu Sirsasana)

All forward bends invite new energy and tone the vital organs of the body. They lengthen and release tightness in the back side of the body. In particular, this pose releases the calves, hamstrings, glutes, and back and improves blood circulation in the legs.

Building Blocks

1. Bring your left heel in to the inside of your right thigh.
2. Keep your right foot active and press the top of your right thigh into the floor.
3. Exhale and reach forward to grab your foot with both hands (or your ankle, if that is better for you).
4. Breathe in and lift halfway up to a straight back, then exhale and fold forward.
5. Gaze down at your extended leg and hold for five breaths.

Alignment

- Keep the foot of the extended leg active.
- Press the top of the extended thigh into the floor.
- Hinge at your hips.
- Pull your belly in and up.
- Relax your face, neck, and eyes.

Connecting Vinyasa

After five breaths, release the foot and come back up to a seated position.

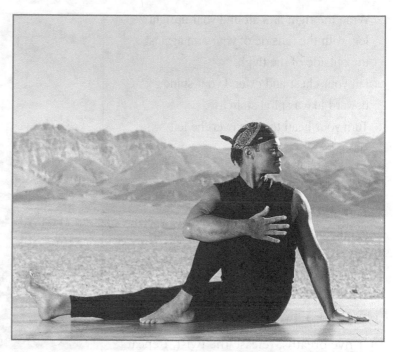

Pose 24: Straight Leg Seated Twist (Parivrtta Marichyasana)

Pose 24: Straight Leg Seated Twist (Parivrtta Narichyasana)

This is a wonderful counterpose for standing poses. It boosts blood flow to the vital body and spine, rinses the lower and middle back, liver, spleen, and kidneys, and stimulates the digestive organs.

Building Blocks

1. Sit with your right leg straight and your left knee bent with the left foot flat on the floor.

If you want to try a little extra twisting action in this pose, work your left ear down toward your right knee as you lift your right ribs up high.

2. Wrap the right arm around your upright leg, with the outside of your arm against the outside of the thigh.
3. Lift your chest and extend your spine upward like a spiral staircase.
4. Turn your head to gaze over the left shoulder.

Alignment

- Activate your thighs and feet.
- On the in breath, lift; on the out breath, twist.
- Relax as you rotate.

Connecting Vinyasa

After five breaths, release the twist. Repeat the sequence of Lifted Leg Pose, Twisting Lifted Leg Pose, Easy Forward Bend, and Straight Leg Seated Twist, this time with the left leg extended. After five breaths in Straight Leg Seated Twist, extend both legs out straight in front of you in preparation for the next pose, Seated Forward Bend.

Pose 25: Seated Forward Bend (Paschimotonasana)

Seated Forward Bend is a wonderful cooling pose that unclutters the mind and leaves you feeling neutral, balanced, and restored.

Building Blocks

1. Straighten your legs out in front of you so they are together with the ankles touching.

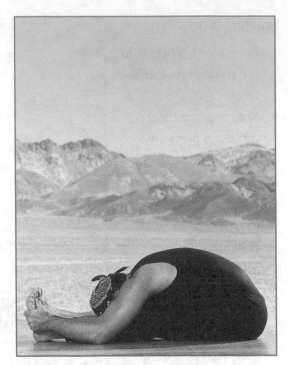

Pose 25: Seated Forward Bend (Paschimotonasana)

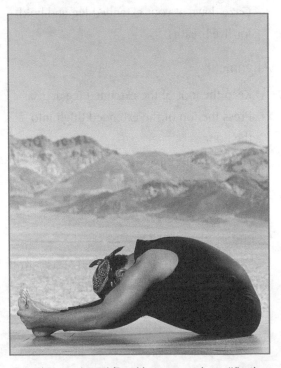

Seated Forward Bend (Paschimotonasana), modification

2. Use your hands to pull your sitting muscles out laterally so you come right onto your sitting bones.
3. Exhale and reach forward, hinging from the hips, and grab your feet, ankles, or legs with both hands.
4. Inhale and lift halfway up to a flat back.
5. Exhale and fold forward.
6. Gaze to your legs for ten breaths.

Alignment

- Flex your feet and press through the balls of the feet.
- Hinge at your hips, not at your waist.
- Press the tops of your thighs down toward the floor.
- Spin your inner thighs downward.
- On the inhalation, use your hands to pull you forward. On the exhalation, draw your torso down toward your knees.
- Relax your shoulders.
- Allow your neck to be neutral and free.
- Melt into the deep release.

Modification

You can bend your knees if you need to if you feel any low back strain. If you can't reach your feet, use a towel or strap around your feet as an extended handle.

Connecting Vinyasa

After the tenth exhalation, inhale and come back up to a seated position. Lie down on your back in preparation for the next pose, Dead Bug.

Pose 26: Dead Bug Pose (Urdhva Mukha Upavista Konasana)

Dead Bug pose gives a final stretch to the hips, hamstrings, and inner thighs, and also releases the lower spine. It slows the heart rate and allows your body to begin to come into a resting state.

Building Blocks

1. From the horizontal prone position, inhale and bring your knees up to your chest.
2. Hold on to the inner edges of your feet, thumbs facing down toward your heels.
3. Very gently, use your hands to pull your feet, knees, and quadriceps toward the floor.
4. Roll your tailbone down toward your mat and lengthen your spine into the floor.

Alignment

- Stack your ankles over your knees.
- Spread your thighs to the outer edges of your torso.

It does not matter how far you reach in the pose. What matters is how you hold it in general: the compassion, intention, and overall integration of your movement.

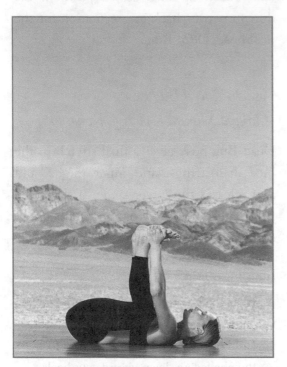

Pose 26: Dead Bug Pose
(Urdhva Mukha Upavista Konasana)

- Pull the soles of your feet downward.
- Move your tailbone down toward the floor.
- Lengthen the line of your spine flat into the floor.
- Allow your belly to drop and soften.

Pose 27: *Savasana*

This final restful pose is the gateway to the deep, meditative state that leads us to the source of infinite wisdom and heart-centered awareness.

Building Blocks/Alignment

1. Lie on your back with your legs straight and separated about twelve inches apart.
2. Allow your feet to relax and splay out.
3. Place your arms alongside your body, about six inches away from you, palms facing up.
4. Roll your shoulder blades in toward each other. This allows your chest to expand and your breathing to shift profoundly.
5. Pull your head out of your neck, your arms out of your shoulders, and your legs out of your hips.
6. Really feel the floor beneath you and your contact to it.
7. Drop your belly.
8. Drop your brain.
9. Release your whole body.
10. Make any last adjustments you need to be comfortable, and just let go.

You've done your part; you've met the universe halfway. Now just relax and let the universe do its part on your behalf.

BARON BAPTISTE

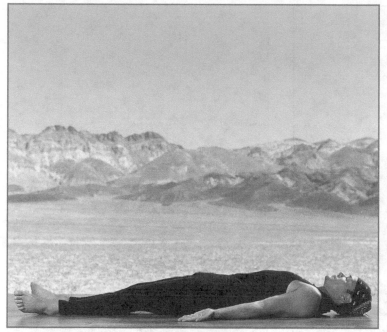

Pose 27: Savasana

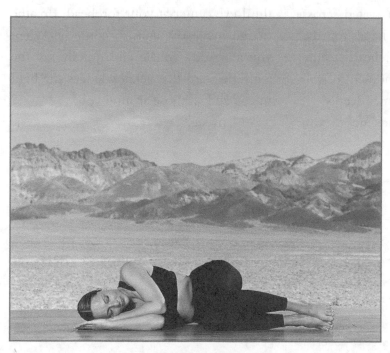

Closing sequence I

Modification

If your lower back hurts, you can bend your knees and set the soles of your feet on the floor. You can also prop your torso up with blankets, or roll one up and place it underneath your knees.

Connecting Vinyasa

Stay here as long as you like. If you can, it is best to rest in Savasana for at least ten minutes. Though this will add to the length of your practice, it is so beneficial to let your nervous system assimilate all the good you have done in your practice.

Closing Your Practice

The following sequence is done at the end of each yoga sequence throughout these forty days. When you are ready and with your eyes closed, roll onto your right side from Savasana and curl up into a little ball. Stay here for as long as feels right, then

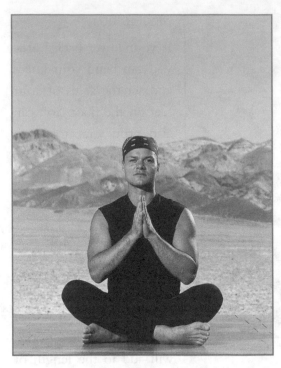

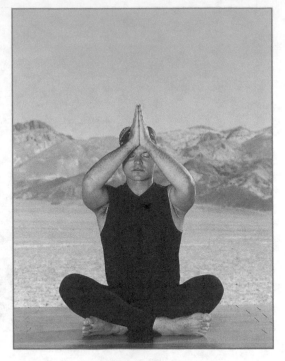

Closing sequence II

Closing sequence III

very slowly come up to a seated, cross-legged position. Bring your hands together in a prayer position at your heart's center and either sit quietly in a moment of stillness or chant "om" three times deeply.

Slowly bring your hands up to your third-eye center at your forehead. Breathe in and invite the light to come in. When you are ready, inhale and quietly say the Sanskrit word that acknowledges the light in you and all those around you:

"Namaste."

For a quick reference to this week's poses, see page 235.

Week One Balancing Diet

Do not wait until one is thirsty before digging a well.

—NEI JING

FOR THOUSANDS OF YEARS, TRADITIONAL CULTURES LOOKED AT THE BODY AS A FUNCTIONING WHOLE. THERE WAS NO SUCH THING AS MIND/BODY MEDICINE OR

practices, because mind and body were never separated in the first place. Ancient societies inherently got it that health embodies the whole person, on every level—attitudes, actions, how they live their lives, and what they eat. Then history marched on, and we divided and industrialized, until we completely turned our backs on the concept of wholeness. In the realm of diet, we have become so obsessed with compartmentalizing our diet into fat, calories, carbs, and so on that we have completely forgotten the most basic of connections: that we are, in essence, what we eat. And, it seems, how we eat it.

When we look at the diets of wealthy countries such as the United States, we find an abundance of excess. We have forgotten the profound wisdom of the Bible: "There are no riches greater than a sound body." We gorge ourselves on supersize sodas and huge portions of calorie-rich fast food, and line our supermarket shelves with rows and rows of processed, fake foods. Everything is available to us in abundance, and that isn't necessarily always a good thing. There is so much excess that we have lost our internal gauge of how much is enough amid the buffet of life. Even recreational activities such as going to the movies turns into a food frenzy, with gallon-size tubs (tubs!) of buttered popcorn and enormous bags of sugary candy. All-you-can-eat buffets, triple cheeseburgers, fried dough balls powdered with sugar and cinnamon that come free with your deep-dish pizza—the excess is all around us, consuming us as we consume it.

As a result of all this, millions of Americans are physically out of balance and suffer from chronic diseases that are directly linked to our diet. We have so distanced ourselves from really getting that what we eat directly affects our bodies, our health, our moods, and our lives, continually stuffing our faces to distract ourselves from feeling the effects. The concept of excess is deeply ingrained in the psyche of our culture, which makes it that much harder to wake up and realize that eating this way just *doesn't make intuitive sense.*

In the first week of your personal revolution program, we are aiming to bring you back into your body so that you can begin to really understand your relationship to food and what your particular body needs. The reason diets don't work is because they assume everyone is the same, but as I said in *Journey into Power,* no one can slap a universal diet on everyone and claim it will work absolutely. We all have different bodies and different requirements.

Based on the very simple categorizations in traditional Chinese medicine, we can begin to understand our own individual body ecology and what foods we need to come back into balance. Why bother seeking balance? Because reaching this state of equilibrium is the real secret to shedding the excess weight and toxins in our bodies. Added pounds, lethargy, and all kinds of other physical symptoms are a result of us being out of balance. We don't need to wait until illness, disease, or obesity happen before we seek balance; we can wake up anytime we are ready.

We all have different body patterns. Being in touch with your individual pattern can help you stay conscious of how you can nourish your particular body to optimal health and vitality. Before you read about the different body patterns, remember that overintellectualizing anything never really helps anyone. In fact, overthinking gets in the way of our natural intuition. If we spend too much time thinking or worrying about what we eat, no matter how healthy, it ruins our enjoyment of food and causes problems in our heads and our bellies. Understanding these patterns can be a great tool, but it is not meant to rule your life. It is simply meant to act as a guideline for you to make changes however you intuitively see fit.

Hot/Cold Body Patterns

Within each of us are the properties of heat and cold. Ideally, our bodies find the right balance between the two, but in our crazy, often unnatural world, that rarely happens. Most of us end up with an excess of heat or cold in our bodies, which manifests as all kinds of physical symptoms, including being under- or overweight, having blood pressure that is too high or too low, and being fatigued, just to name a few. We all experience different levels of heat and cold in the body at different times, but the idea is to discover which end of the continuum applies more to your life. Realizing where you fall on the continuum helps you make slow, long-term changes in what you eat, because as you'll see, the basic categories of hot and cold can also easily be applied to all foods.

People with an excess of heat generally dislike hot weather. They like cold beverages in quantity, sweat easily, and have difficulty sleeping. These people may have loud voices and skin prone to breakouts. Heat-excessive individuals may also be irritable and/or have a bad temper.

Those with an excess of cold generally dislike cold weather. They like warm or hot beverages in sips, do not sweat easily, and curl up when sleeping. They may have soft voices and pale skin. Those who are cold-excessive are usually quiet and reserved in nature.

Our bodies are always in flux in terms of hot and cold, depending on the season and on what is going on for and within us at any given time. So because you might be heat-deficient right now does *not* mean

Foods That Are More Heating	Foods That Are More Cooling
Calorie-rich foods	Lighter food, such as salads
Dense meat: lamb, beef, turkey, chicken, pork	Less dense meat: white fish, shellfish, clams, crab
Bread, rice, and other grains (because of their high caloric content)	Soy products
Nuts (high caloric content)	Dairy products
Chiles	Most types of beans
Ginger	Cucumbers
Garlic	Peppermint
Onions	Broccoli
Peppers	Bok choy
Mustard greens	Kale
Coffee	Celery
Cinnamon	Green tea
Alcohol (ideally cutting back)	Yogurt
	Watermelon

that you will be heat-deficient forever. This isn't about casting you into one fixed body type. We are always on a continuum between opposites; like a boat on the water, we rock from one side to the other, finding balance for a split second in between. In time, the alternations become less extreme and we are much more easily able to intuit what we need and when.

Just as our bodies hold heat or cold, so do foods. As you intuitively start to understand whether your body needs to be cooled or warmed to come back into balance, you can choose foods that will have the desired effect. If we remember that a calorie is a degree of heat, then it makes sense that the more calories a food has, the more heat it produces. Examples of foods that have a heating quality are meat, starchy vegetables, and cooked foods with a liberal use of spices. The fewer the calories, the more cooling a food is. Cooling foods are generally ones that are lighter in nature, such as raw vegetables or fruit juices.

Deficient/Excessive Body Patterns

Just as we are always in a cycle between hot and cold, our bodies are also always in ei-

Foods That Cleanse	Foods That Build
Smaller portions of any food	Bigger portions of all foods
Water-based vegetables	All whole grains
Water-based fruits	Starchy food
Carrots	All processed, refined, additive-filled
Dandelion greens	foods (ideally cutting back)
Salads	Milk and milk products
Seaweeds	Root vegetables such as potatoes and
Fruit juice	yams
Soups	Soy milk
Tomato sauce	Whey
Spices—ginger, cumin, cardamom,	Pasta
peppermint	Oatmeal
Fish, such as sardines, that are not so	Oils
dense	Dense meats such as beef, lamb, and
	pork

ther in the building phase of a cycle or the cleansing phase. When we need to build, we are in a state of *deficiency*. When we need to cleanse, we are in a state of *excess*. We need to build whenever we feel any combination of: weak, depleted, run-down, thin, fragile, anxious without knowing why, having a sensation of something lacking. In contrast, we need to cleanse whenever we feel any combination of: overweight, an accumulation of toxins, sluggishness, fogginess in the head, overburdened.

I usually go through a few cycles of cleansing and building throughout the year, and I've come to appreciate the Chinese medicine practitioners' wisdom that the needs of our bodies change according to the seasons. Generally, I build in the summer, cleanse in the fall, build in the winter, then cleanse again in the spring. That is what has felt right to me; in time you, too, will find the rhythm that feels right to you.

It is fairly easy to intuit what kinds of foods cleanse and what kinds of foods build. Those that cleanse are water-rich and light, and the ones that build are nutrient-dense and more substantial. Take a look at the chart above to get a sense of which foods fall where on the continuum.

Week One Diet To-Do

Identify yourself in the basic patterns of hot or cold, excessive or deficient, remembering that you may not have all the qualities of one specific pattern. The idea is to find the one that most closely describes you. Then start to incorporate some of the foods that your body needs into your diet, whether they are warming, cooling, cleansing, or building.

You don't have to overhaul your entire diet all at once—that is using the brute force of your will, and as we all know, willpower does not work. If you start to make the changes in smaller chunks, at whatever pace feels intuitively right for you, I believe you will rediscover a sense of rightful balance that lets the excess weight, toxicity, and lethargy melt away. Then it becomes less about struggling to give up your cravings and bad habits, and more about letting them give you up.

One thing that will help support making these changes is your daily yoga practice. Your mat becomes a mirror, and as you step onto it every morning, you will be able to start seeing the direct effects of your diet. As the week goes by, you will really start to come back into your body—to see and feel and understand on a deep and personal level the connection between what you feed your body and how it feels and performs.

Week One Presence Meditation

5 Minutes

MEDITATION CULTIVATES PRESENCE. THE MECHANICS OF AWARENESS-BASED MEDITATION IN-VOLVE AIMING THE MIND AND SUSTAINING YOUR AWARENESS ON AN

object. It is much like picking up a string bean with a fork. You would need to spear it just deeply enough in order to lift it off the plate into your mouth. To do this you need two things: *right aim* and *right energy*. Without right aim, you would just swing your fork around and miss the string bean every time. Instead, you take aim and pick up the targeted bean. If you are too forceful, you'll mash the bean and maybe even break the plate; if you are too passive, the fork will fall right out of your hand. Right aim and right energy are essential principles in meditation that can be applied to almost anything.

This week in meditation we'll focus on the act of being present. We'll aim our mind directly to the moment at hand, and apply just the right amount of energy to our breath. We focus our mind and our non-forceful energy on the ebb and flow of our breath, but only on the breath that is right here in this moment. *Just this one breath.* Have no concern for the breath that came before it or the one that will follow. Just one breath at a time. Remember each time you drift off into your thoughts to re-aim and begin again.

Sit this way for at least five minutes each morning and five minutes every night before you go to bed.

1. How much am I taking responsibility to learn and grow from the experiences, both easy and difficult, that I have in my life?

2. What are my beliefs about:

   • My body? (Do I believe it is "too heavy," "too weak," or just right? Do I believe it serves me well?)

   • My relationships? (Do they nourish me? What purpose do they serve in my growth and my life? Do I believe I am treated as I want or ought to be?)

   • My work? (Is it fulfilling?)

   • Spirituality? (Do I believe in a higher power?)

   • Sex? (What role does it play in my life? Do I experience shame or joy around it? Do I misuse it? Do I see it as a vehicle for spiritual and emotional expression?)

   • Money? (Do I believe it is it the root of all evil, or does it simply give me freedom to do what I want in life? Do I have a lot of fear around making it or keeping it?)

3. When in my life am I fully present? In my job? With my partner or kids? When I am working? When I am playing? When I am alone?

4. Where in my life am I hiding? In other words, where do I privately know that I need to take more responsibility and/or become fully present?

5. Where in my life am I flirting with disaster?

Week Two: Vitality

THERE IS A BELIEF IN OUR CULTURE THAT WE HAVE TO GET AWAY OR GO SOMEPLACE EXOTIC IN ORDER TO REJUVENATE AND REDISCOVER OUR LOST RADIANCE. YET I

believe vitality is something we can find right here, within each moment of our lives. It doesn't need to be something we taste for only a few days on vacation and then disappears. Vitality is very simply an energy that comes from living a life of enlightened knowledge and action. When we do what we know to be right and true, we are revitalized and renewed right where we live.

There once was a young prince named Siddhartha, who later in life became the Buddha. One day he decided to go off into the mountains and seek truth, inner transformation, and spiritual vitality. This

search for enlightenment meant leaving all that he was and owned: his kingdom, his parents, his wife, and his child. Although he was full of doubts about his journey, he made up his mind and snuck out in the middle of the night without telling anyone.

After twelve years, he became an enlightened man. In his new radiance, he returned to his palace to apologize to those he loved for leaving. The first person he encountered was his father, who was very angry. For an hour, his father chewed him out and attempted to shame him for abandoning his crown, his family, and his responsibility. The father was ranting and raving when suddenly he stopped and noticed that his son, the Buddha, was just standing there in perfect composure and peace, completely unaffected.

The Buddha said, "This is what I wanted for you, Father. I wanted you to get all that off your chest. Please dry your tears and really look at me, because I am not the same boy who left the palace twelve years ago. Your son died a long time ago. I look like your son, but my whole being has changed. I am a new man."

"I can see you have changed," the father replied. "You were at one time so hot-tempered and reactive, yet now you had no response to my anger toward you."

Then the Buddha's wife approached him and said, "I can see that you have been transformed, but these last twelve years have been really sad for me. You have obviously changed; you radiate a different light. Your presence is totally new and fresh; your eyes are pure and clear.

"However," she went on to say, "I have one question for you. This transformation—this new enlightened way of being that you have attained—could you not have attained it right here at home in your palace? Did your home and family somehow prevent you from finding truth and transformation?"

"I could have done it right here at home," the Buddha responded, "but in my ignorance, I did not know that. There was no need to go to the mountains, no need for me to go anywhere. I had to go inside myself, and that could have happened anywhere."

Your practice this week is all about revealing the vitality in your own life, right here, where you are. In Week Two, your yoga practice will increase to thirty minutes and will enable you to taste the energy of vitality on a physical level. We will introduce the concept of fresh, life-giving foods into your Balancing Diet, and the focus of your meditation will be noticing and releasing the self-damaging tapes that run in your head and block your vitality. The excavation questions will open your eyes to the practices and behaviors in your life that are blocking your natural vitality and radiance from shining through.

Week Two Yoga Practice
30 Minutes

NOW THAT YOU HAVE MANY OF THE INITIAL POSES HARDWIRED INTO YOUR NERVOUS SYSTEM,

WE'LL INCREASE OUR DAILY PRACTICE TIME BY TEN MINUTES. YOU AL-

ready know the basics of many of these poses, so your flow will most likely become more fluid and natural.

Beginning Vinyasa

As in the first week of practice, open with the three integration poses: Child's Pose (1), Downward Facing Dog (2), and Ragdoll (3). Then do two rounds of Sun Salutation A and two rounds of Sun Salutation B. After the second round of Sun Salutation B, go through the steps of Sun Salutation B only up until Warrior I with your right foot forward.

Pose 4: Warrior II

From Warrior I, move into Warrior II (see p. 79 for building blocks and alignment). IIold Warrior II for five breaths.

Pose 5: Reverse Warrior

After five breaths in Warrior II, drop your left arm down to your back leg and take Reverse Warrior (p. 80). Hold for five breaths.

Connecting Vinyasa

After five breaths, come back up to Warrior II. This puts you in position for the next pose, Triangle.

Pose 6: Triangle (Trikonasana)

Triangle Pose allows you to open up and infuse life through your whole body, working out any kinks or compressions. It allows you to be expansive in your body.

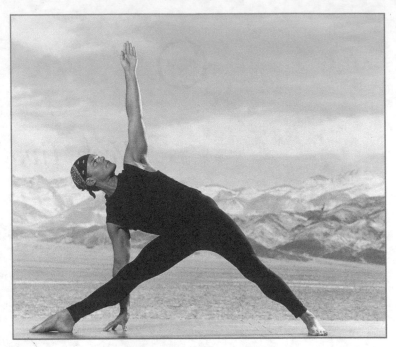

Pose 6: Triangle Pose (Trikonasana)

Building Blocks

1. From Warrior II, straighten your front leg on track.
2. With straight legs, press your left thigh back and reach toward the front wall with your right hand, bringing your torso over your front thigh.
3. Reach down and grab your left shin (or ankle, or the floor, whichever is best for you).
4. Float your left arm up to the sky.

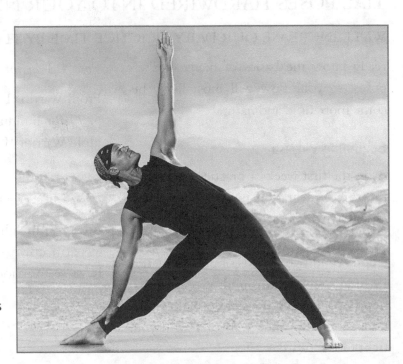

Triangle Pose (Trikonasana), modification

Concentrate on dropping the lower side of your rib cage toward the floor, stacking your upper lung over the lower. This will keep your torso rotating up and give you full expression through your whole upper body.

5. Gaze high at your upper hand and take five deep breaths.

Alignment

- Keep your heels on one line.
- Maintain strong, active legs.
- Spiral your inner thighs outward, away from each other.
- Scoop your tailbone down and under.
- Pull your tail in and pull your belly in so you are on one plane.
- Stack your right hand over your right shoulder.
- Lengthen your spine.
- Draw your scapula down.
- Keep your upper hand active.

Modification

Place your hand on your shin, just below your kneecap. If you feel any strain in your neck, bring your chin to your lower shoulder.

Connecting Vinyasa

After five breaths in Triangle, inhale and let your raised arm pull you back up to standing. Bend your front knee into Warrior II, windmill your hands down to the mat, and step back to High Push-Up. Go through Sun Salutation B again, ending in Warrior I, then repeat Warrior II, Reverse Warrior, and Triangle with your left leg forward. After the final breath in Triangle, go through Vinyasa A (High to Low Push-Up, Upward Facing Dog, Downward Facing Dog), ending in Downward Facing Dog.

Pose 7: Side Plank (Vasisthasana)

Side Plank is a dynamic pose that helps build tremendous purifying heat. It tones and strengthens your arms and torso, and trains all the muscles in your body to work as one integrated force.

Building Blocks

1. From Downward Facing Dog, move your torso forward and drop your hips down, coming back into High Push-Up position.
2. Bring your feet together so your inner ankles and thighs are touching.
3. Spin your heels to the right, coming onto the outside edge of your right foot.
4. Float your left arm up to the sky.
5. Gaze to the thumbnail of your upper hand.

Alignment

- Stack your upper hip directly over the lower one.

- Keep your heels, hips, and heart all in one line.
- Draw your tailbone down toward your heels.
- Lift your hips high.
- Align your upper arm above your lower arm, stacking all the joints along one plane.
- Drop your shoulder blades down your back, away from your ears.
- Open your chest.

Modification

If you want, you can drop your lower knee to the floor directly underneath your hip and spin your upper foot flat so the sole of your foot presses into the floor. In this variation, your right hand, knee, and back foot should all be in one line.

Connecting Vinyasa

After five breaths, roll open a little more and then come back to High Push-Up position. Go through Vinyasa A until you come to Downward Facing Dog.

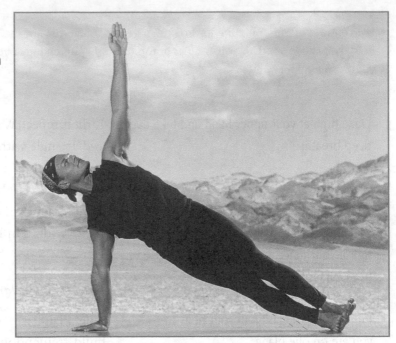

Pose 7: Side Plank (Vasisthasana)

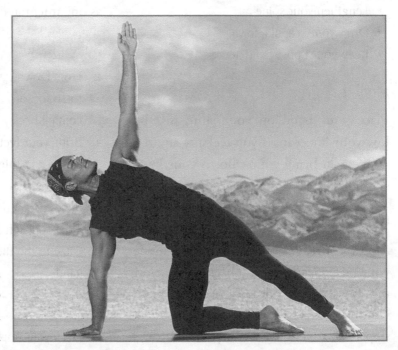

Side Plank (Vasisthasana), modification

You don't want to jam all your body weight onto your lower wrist. Engage all the muscles in your body to stabilize and energize this pose. Flex your feet, contract your legs, activate your abdominal lock; pull your arms away from each other, and pull the crown of your head and the soles of your feet apart, to create full-body length and traction.

Pose 8: Crescent Lunge (Anjaneyasana)

Crescent Lunge is another dynamic, full-body pose that integrates all your muscles. It creates flexible strength and stability in the lower body and a beautiful, fluid length through the upper body.

Building Blocks

1. From Downward Facing Dog, look up and step your right foot forward to your right hand, bending your front knee to 90 degrees.
2. Leave your back heel up so you are standing on the ball of your back foot.
3. Tuck your tail under.
4. Inhale and sweep your arms up over your head with your palms facing each other.
5. Exhale and bring your arms down, holding your hands together in a prayerlike position at your chest with your palms pressing together.
6. Fuse your gaze to a point in front of you.

Alignment

- Face both feet forward and press through the balls of your feet.
- You should have about four inches between your feet. If your feet are on one line, you will have trouble balancing.

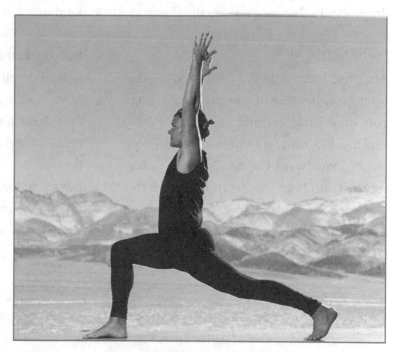

Pose 8: Crescent Lunge (Anjaneyasana)

- Pull your right hip back and your left hip forward, squaring your hips so they face the wall in front of you.
- Maintain a strong, straight, and very active back leg.
- Lift your back knee and quadriceps toward the ceiling.
- Stack your front knee over your ankle; keep moving it out toward the baby toe.
- Contract your abdomen to stabilize your core.
- Soften your front ribs down toward your belly.
- Reach up through the crown of your head to create upper body length.

Modification

To reduce the intensity of this movement, drop your back knee down to the floor.

Connecting Vinyasa

After five breaths, lower your hands to the floor on either side of your front foot. Step your foot back, coming into High Push-Up (8). Go through Vinyasa A until you are in Downward Facing Dog (2). Come forward into High Push-Up and repeat the sequence of Side Plank and Crescent Lunge on the left side. From the second Crescent Lunge, go through Vinyasa A

again, ending in Standing Forward Bend (6). From Standing Forward Bend, take Thunderbolt, which will lead directly into the next pose, Prayer Twist.

Pose 9: Prayer Twist
(Parivrtta Utkatasana)

Prayer Twist is a powerful way to detoxify the organs and glands in the midbody.

Building Blocks

1. From Thunderbolt, reach up through your hands, and as you exhale, bring them down into a prayerlike position at your heart center. Inhale here.
2. Exhale and spin your left elbow to the outside of your right thigh.
3. Keep your feet together and dip your hips low.
4. Pull your butt back and your chest plate forward, lengthening your spine.
5. Now, straighten your arms, setting your lower hand in a claw to the outside of your right foot and your right arm straight up to the sky.
6. Bring your lower shoulder blade forward and your upper shoulder blade back.
7. Gaze to your upper hand and breathe for five.

Work your twist by lengthening the spine on the inhalation and twisting your torso open on the exhalation. Match your breath to each micromovement.

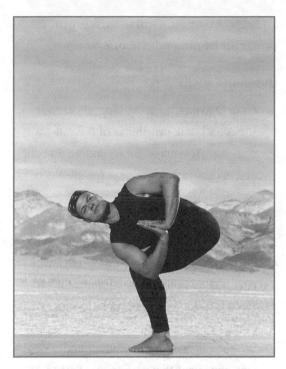

Pose 9: Prayer Twist (Parivrtta Utkatasana), step 1

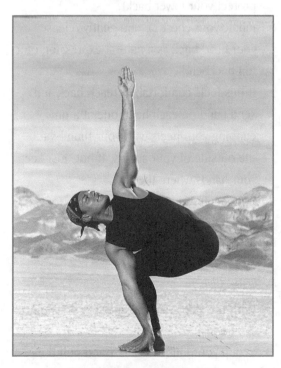

Prayer Twist (Parivrtta Utkatasana), step 2

Alignment

- Keep your feet together.
- Maintain strong legs.
- Keep your knees level and together.
- Squeeze your sitting bones and inner thighs in toward each other.
- Press your hips/tail back and pull your chest forward.
- Twist from your torso, not your arms.
- Stack your upper hand directly above your shoulder.

Connecting Vinyasa

After five breaths, relax forward into Ragdoll (3). Relax for a few breaths, then bend your knees to come back into Thunderbolt. Bring your hands to namaste and take Prayer Twist to the left side. After five breaths on the left side, relax forward into Ragdoll once again. Take a few breaths in Ragdoll, then come rolling back up to Samasthiti. Go through Vinyasa A, ending in Downward Facing Dog. From Downward Facing Dog, lower your knees to the mat in preparation for the next pose, Camel.

Pose 10: Camel Pose (Ustrasana)

Camel Pose is the reverse position of sitting. It is a back-bending pose that helps undo all the tightness in the hips, psoas, and some of the rotator muscles, which affect the entire body's ability to move. Camel pose also opens the heart center,

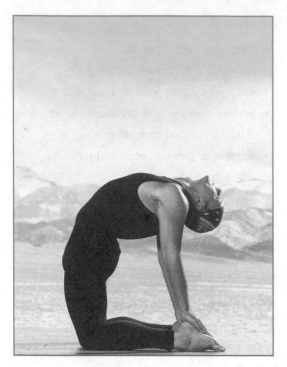

Pose 10: Camel (Ustrasana)

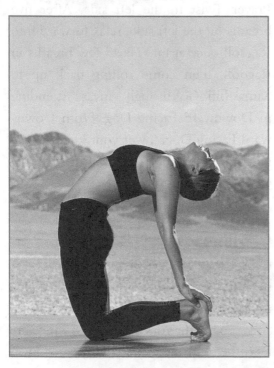

Camel (Ustrasana), modification

and for many students, this promotes a powerful healing release of emotions.

Building Blocks

1. From Downward Facing Dog, drop your knees and walk two-thirds of the way up your mat. You may want to double up your mat underneath your knees for a little extra padding.
2. Stand up on your knees.
3. Separate your knees and feet to hip width.
4. Bring your hands to your lower back with your fingers pointing up, thumbs into your sacrum. Wrap your elbows in towards each other.
5. Scoop your tailbone down and under (it is *very* important that you do this first to protect your lower back).
6. Inhale your chest up and gently release your head back as a natural expression of a full backbend.
7. If this feels comfortable, reach back and set a hand on each heel, one at a time, cupping your heels with your thumbs to the outside of your ankles. If not, just keep your hands where they are.
8. Soften your face and set your eyes to a spot behind you.
9. Hold for five breaths.

Alignment

- Root the shins, ankles, and feet down into the floor.
- Scoop your tailbone under and pull the front of your pelvis upward.

If you can't swallow comfortably in this pose, your neck is at risk. To ensure your neck is in a stable position, first pull your chin back into your neck, as though you were holding a pencil in the crease between your chin and neck. *Then* slowly lower your head back.

- Engage your abdominal lock.
- Engage your lower body, making it very strong.
- Press your hips forward until the thighs are vertical.
- Lift your chest up high to the sky as you press down in your lower body.
- Drop your shoulder blades down your back.

Modification

If this feels too intense on your lower back, curl your toes under and stand on the balls of your feet.

Connecting Vinyasa

After the five breaths, tuck your chin to your chest, squeeze your lower body and root down, and from that leg strength slowly float back up so you are standing on your shins. Come into Downward Facing Dog (2) for five breaths, then repeat Camel a second time. End in Downward Facing Dog. After five breaths, come down to your hands and knees, cross your feet, and roll over your ankles to lie down on your back.

Pose 11: Bridge Pose (Setubandasana)

Bridge Pose continues the back-bending release, opening the chest and stretching the abdominal wall. It also preps the soil of our bodies for Wheel.

Building Blocks

1. Lie on your back and place your feet flat on the floor at hip width, knees over your heels (not over the toes).

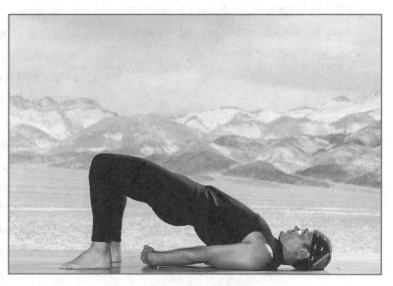

Pose 11: Bridge Pose (Setubandasana)

2. Tilt your pelvis and scoop your tailbone under.

3. Inhale and lift your hips up high, coming onto your shoulders.

4. Walk your shoulder blades in toward each other underneath your torso and clasp your hands together, interlacing your fingers.

5. Press down through your feet and upper arms as you lift your hips up high.

6. Set your eyes on the tip of your nose.

Alignment

- Feet are hip width and parallel (or slightly splayed for more comfort in your knees).
- Stack your knees over your ankles. Do not let them splay out to the sides.
- Spin your inner thighs down toward the floor.
- Press down through the soles and lift your hips high.
- On the in breath, expand your rib cage; on the out breath, drive the feet and upper arms down and the hips higher.

Modification

If you cannot lift your hips up high, just do what you can. Work to your capacity, even if that means coming up only a few inches.

Connecting Vinyasa

After five breaths, release your hands and lower your hips to your mat. Take two deep breaths.

Pose 12: Wheel
(Urdhva Dhanurasana)

Wheel is one of the most powerful poses in yoga practice. It unfolds the entire front side of the body while strengthening and conditioning the entire back side. This is one of the best poses to open and release tension in the upper back, chest, shoulders, and hip flexors, as well as the lower back. It also opens the heart center and can create tremendous emotional release.

Building Blocks

Step One

1. Lie on your back with your knees up, feet flat on the floor at hip width.

2. Place your hands flat next to your ears with the palms down and your fingertips facing toward your shoulders.

3. Draw your elbows in so they are in line with your shoulder joints, and drop your shoulders down toward your buttocks.

4. Exhale and scoop your tail under.

5. Inhale and press down through the soles of your feet and hands, coming onto the crown of your head. If this is far as you can go, stay here, taking care to put your body weight into your hands and arms rather than your neck. If you feel you can straighten your arms and come up, move on to Step Two.

6. Once again, draw your elbows in so they are in line with your shoulder joints and slide your shoulder blades down your back. *It is very important that you do this before coming up to prevent shoulder damage.*

7. Exhale here.

8. On the inhalation, press down through the soles of your feet and hands and straighten your arms, launching up into a beautiful back bend.

9. Let your head hang heavy and your neck be free.

10. Relax your face and gaze to a spot on the wall behind you.

Alignment

- Feet are parallel or slightly splayed.
- Root your four limbs down and press your hips up.
- Spin your inner thighs down toward the floor.

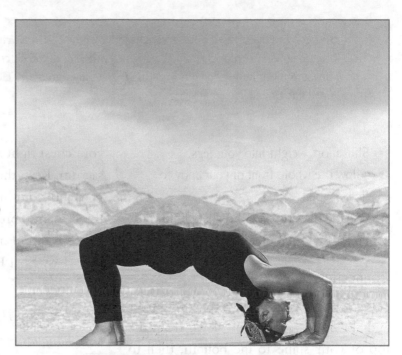

Pose 12: Wheel (Urdhva Dhanurasana), step 1, preparation

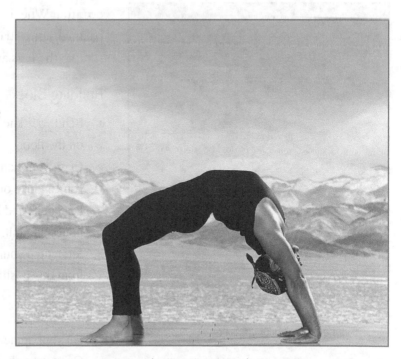

Wheel (Urdhva Dhanurasana), step 2

- Shift more weight into your legs.
- Allow the whole front of your body to flower open.
- Use the power of your breath to hold you up for the count of five.

Connecting Vinyasa

After five breaths, tuck your chin under and slowly lower yourself down from the top of your spine to the bottom, then to your hips. Do not draw your knees into your chest right away; this will shock your sacrum. Keep the soles of your feet on the mat and your hips down. Rest here for three to five breaths, then come up to a seated position in preparation for the next pose, Easy Boat Pose.

Pose 13: Easy Boat Pose (Sukhanavasana)

Easy Boat Pose is simply a supported/modified version of Boat Pose, which I like to do after Wheel. It develops coordination, balance, and structural integrity, and also sculpts the legs and abdominals.

Building Blocks

1. Bend your knees and place your feet flat on the floor.
2. Clasp your hands behind your knees (or you can take one hand to one wrist).
3. Lean back and balance on your sitting bones and tail.
4. Straighten your legs as much as you can from this position.

Alignment

- Lift your spine.
- Open your chest.

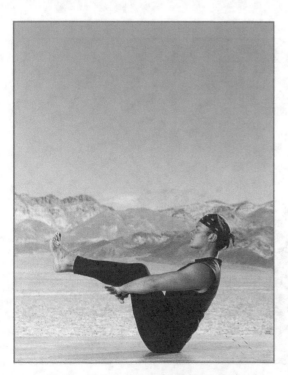

Pose 13: Easy Boat Pose (Sukhanavasana)

- Fan your toes and feet.
- Soften the muscles in your face; a hint of a smile is always nice.

Connecting Vinyasa

After five breaths, lower your feet back to the floor and unclasp your hands. From there, you will go right into regular Boat Pose, below.

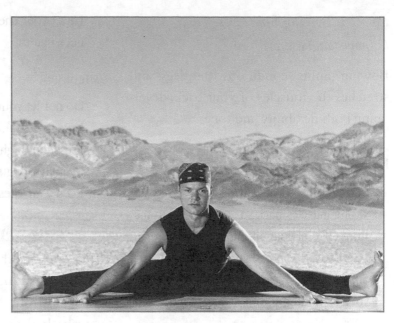

Pose 15: Sitting Splits Pose (Urdhvakonasana)

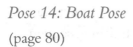

Pose 14: Boat Pose
(page 80)

Take Boat Pose five times, crossing your legs and lifting your body off the ground each time in between, as you did in Week One.

Connecting Vinyasa

After the fifth repetition, end in a seated position. With your legs spread wide to each side, set your hands firmly into the floor and lift your chest, activating your thighs and feet.

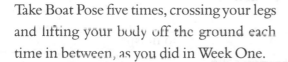

Pose 15: Sitting Splits Pose (Urdhvakonasana)

Sitting Splits Pose opens the hips, releases and lengthens the inner thighs and hamstrings, and stabilizes and strengthens the lower back. It also serves as preparation

and modification for the next pose, Bowing Splits.

Building Blocks

1. From the seated position, extend your legs straight and spread them out wide to each side.
2. Spread your hands firmly into the floor at shoulder width distance apart in front of you.
3. Lift your chest.
4. Gaze forward for five breaths.

Alignment

- Activate your thighs and feet.
- Open your chest.
- Keep your spine elongated.
- Maintain fluid, deep breathing.

Pose 16: Bowing Splits Pose (Upavistakonasana)

Bowing Splits conditions the legs and stretches the muscles of your back, developing both flexibility and tone.

Building Blocks

1. Sitting with your legs wide apart, pull your sitting muscles back so you come onto the front edge of your sitting bones.
2. Lean forward, spread your fingers apart, and walk your hands forward, bringing your torso out in front of you or toward the floor.
3. Move forward until you feel you've reached your edge, then stop.
4. Lower your chest and head, keeping your neck neutral.

Alignment

- Do not let your legs splay inward; your kneecaps should face the ceiling.
- Press the thighs down into the floor.
- Maintain length through your spine.
- Keep your chest broad.

Connecting Vinyasa

After five breaths, slowly work your way back up to sitting, then bring your legs together in front of you. Lower down onto your back, flat on your mat, in preparation for the first pose in the finishing sequence, Dead Bug.

To finish:

Pose 17: Dead Bug Pose (page 89)

Hold Dead Bug for five breaths, then hug your knees into your chest and stay here in preparation for the next pose.

Pose 18: Supine Twist

As a final pose, this twist rinses away any remaining tension, integrating everything you've done by bal-

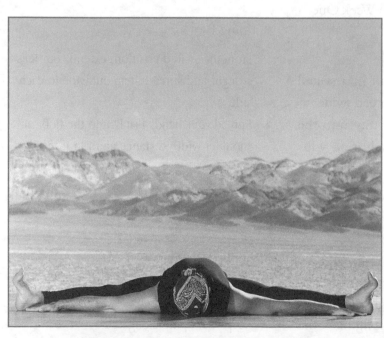

Pose 16: Bowing Splits Pose (Upavistakonasana)

ancing and releasing you on every level.

Building Blocks

1. Straighten your left leg to the floor and pull your right knee in to your chest.
2. Exhale and drop your right knee over to the outer left side of your body.
3. Open your right arm out like a wing and look over your right shoulder.
4. Place your left hand on your right knee.
5. On the inhalation, breathe in purifying air. On the exhalation, breathe away any remaining tension.
6. Close your eyes and just surrender to deep rest.

Alignment

- Create one long, straight line from the crown of your head to the sole of your extended foot.
- Twist to the point that feels good.
- Keep both shoulders on the mat.

Connecting Vinyasa

After five breaths, bring your right leg back to center. Reverse your legs and take another five breaths with your left leg out

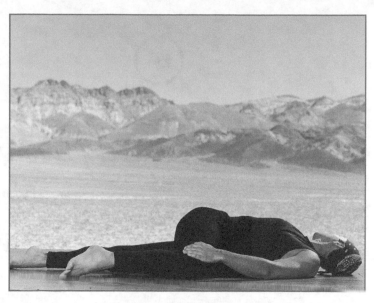

Pose 18: Supine Twist

straight. Return to center, hug your knees into your chest, and then release both legs down to the floor.

Pose 19: Savasana (page 90)

Stay in Savasana for as long as you like.

End by rolling over onto your right side, bringing your hands to your third eye center, breathing deep, and inviting the light as you say, "Namaste."

For a quick reference to this weeks poses, see page 236.

Week Two Balancing Diet

The earth bringeth forth fruit of herself.

—LUKE 4:28

THE NUTRITIONAL EQUIVALENT OF VITAL-
ITY IS FRESH FOOD. IF YOU'VE EVER BEEN TO A CHINA-
TOWN IN ANY PART OF THE WORLD, OR ANY OTHER TRADITIONAL

market, you'll notice that the emphasis is on foods that are healthy, crisp, clean, and life-giving, whether it be fruit, vegetables, or animal products. It's out there in its natural, unprocessed form: whole fish slung into baskets on ice; heaps of fresh, vibrant vegetables piled up; tender, colorful fruit stacked neatly into place.

In contrast, when you walk into a typical grocery store in any town in this country, there are mostly packaged, canned, refined, and frozen foods. Sometimes I walk through the aisles and wonder how we have gone so astray. Frozen meals stacked up advertising healthy this and

low-fat that, bright and enticing packages with limp, processed food inside—it all seems so empty and lifeless. How did we get so far removed from real, whole foods?

I'll tell you how. Food in this country is sold and distributed according to an economy based on shelf life. Everything is created according to how long it will last, how long we can keep it in our cupboards before we have to consume it. This is all very convenient for us and lucrative for the manufacturers, but we pay dearly for it in actual nutrition. For instance, most of the minerals in whole grains are stripped in the process of refinement, which manufacturers do so that the products will last longer. So we get white flour products—what I call "white death"—in the form of breads, cookies, and pastas that may taste good and have a phenomenal shelf life, but absolutely no life at all in terms of nutrition. The canned soups and sauces we buy that are easy and convenient cut down on cooking time, but they also cut down on nutritional value because of all the salt and additives used to preserve them. These chemicals accumulate as toxins in our bodies. Our bodies have no mechanism to process all these alien substances, and so we end up with all kinds of diseases.

When we do our yoga practice the first night of bootcamp, the sweat in the room smells very thick—it's almost as though a cloud of toxicity is hanging in the air as the impurities are coming up and out through the students' pores. The physical rocks of poison are slowly rising to the surface of their gardens to be removed. But as the week progresses and people replace their chemical-laden, heavy diets with foods that are fresh and clean, the smell in the room becomes much, much cleaner and sweeter. I always tell my students that if they don't like the way they smell, they need to change their diet!

Whenever we talk about food and nutrition at bootcamp or workshops, there is always at least one person who says that his or her life is too hectic to be able to buy and prepare fresh food. It does take a bit

more time, but this comes back to your singleness of mind: your commitment. If time is an issue, then be creative and discover ways to make fresh food fast.

In reality, it takes very little time to prepare fresh food. Yes, we have to do a little more than ripping open cellophane packaging and pressing buttons on the microwave, but really, not that much more. Leafy green vegetables such as kale take less than fifteen minutes to prepare and cook. Fresh fish takes six minutes to broil; it takes less than twenty seconds to wash an apple. It may take a few minutes longer to find healthy meals and snacks rather than ordering pizza or dumping quarters into the nearest vending machine, but you end up getting those minutes back later, because you'll live longer.

Throughout this week, take the time to prepare fresh food, and you will realize that it does not have to be a sacrifice. In fact, it can be a joy. We are so lucky to be able to touch and prepare fresh food, so fortunate that it is easily and readily available to us. Even as recently as Gandhi's time, fresh vegetables and fruits were considered delicacies meant only for wealthy city people. When we rush through preparing this kind of food, we create a disconnection between us and what we eat. Chopping vegetables in a food processor may be more convenient than using a knife, but the soulful connection you create between you and the food of God's green earth is so worth the extra five minutes. The conscious care and energy you put into preparing your food comes back to you tenfold. Think about it: Doesn't food prepared with love always taste better than food made in a hurry?

In Week Two, your focus is to fan the purifying flame within and return to a natural state of vibrancy and vitality, and your diet is a key element of this. In this week, you are going to focus your food choices on fresh food. Not canned, not refined, not packaged, not frozen, not microwavable, and most importantly, not from a drive-thru! We're going to focus on *food*, not *food products*—food in its natural and whole form, as it comes to us from the earth.

Week Two Diet To-Do

Make fresh foods the focus of your diet this week. As often as you can, incorporate whole fruits, vegetables, lean meats, fish, and whole grains into your diet. Prepare them in simple ways, with as few added ingredients as possible, to wholly appreciate their natural taste. As the poet Horace observed, "The chief pleasure in eating does not consist in costly seasoning, or exquisite flavor, but in yourself."

As you prepare your food, think about the physical route the food you are eating has taken to get to you. I once saw a news segment about kids in an inner-city school. The reporter asked them where the milk and eggs they ate came from, and they said, "The supermarket." It was so sad to see that they had no idea of its origins before it landed on the grocery store shelf. Where is your food from? Who do you imagine picked it? How did it get to you? This will help you form a closer connection to your food, which is important. Like the Native Americans who gave thanks to the animals who gave their lives to provide food, you will gain a deeper appreciation for the whole cycle of growth, life, and nourishment.

> There is a difference between health food and wholesome food. Health food is fresh, and it mostly cleanses and enlivens. Wholesome food, on the other hand, may be a sugar cookie from Grandma at a holiday meal. It doesn't necessarily cleanse, but it does comfort and nourish us on another level. Moving forward, we need to find ways to marry these two more and more. It's all a balance of proportions, and of feeding ourselves on all levels.

Week Two Vitality Meditation
10 Minutes

WE ALL HAVE TAPES RUNNING IN OUR HEADS THAT TELL US WE AREN'T SMART ENOUGH, GOOD ENOUGH, THIN ENOUGH; THAT WE NEED TO PLEASE PEOPLE; that we should worry; that we have no choice but to obsess, be angry, be resentful, or be fearful. These tapes are programs and conditioning from our past, and holding on to them robs us of our vitality and energy.

As you sit this week, can you create a touch-and-go awareness of the top ten tapes that run in your head? Like the top ten hits on the radio that are played over and over, can you start to notice and gently label the most common themes that play in your mind? It may help to use labels, like "the victim tape," "the worrier tape," "the people-pleaser tape," "the blame tape." Don't judge yourself with these labels; just use them lightheartedly to recognize the patterns that loop in your mind, and then let them go. In this practice, learn to meet these tapes with an open heart.

Do this practice for ten minutes each morning and ten each evening, and in time you will start to notice how draining listening to these tapes can be and how much more vitality you experience when you let them fade away.

Vitality Excavation Questions

1. What is my most meaningful creation in life? Is it my work, my family, myself?

2. What is my most courageous act? Courage doesn't always mean heroism—often courage can show up in more subtle ways, such as having the courage to leave a toxic relationship, to try something you've never done before, or to take a different path than those around you.

3. When do I feel the most energized? For some people, it is when they are working or playing; for others, it is when they are quiet and alone. When do you feel the most alive?

4. What are the forces in my life that drain my energy?

5. Whom do I resent, and how is that resentment affecting me?

Week Three: Equanimity

THERE IS A FAMOUS QUOTE BY THE THEO-
LOGIAN REINHOLD NIEBUHR THAT SAYS, "GOD, GIVE US
THE GRACE TO ACCEPT WITH SERENITY THE THINGS THAT CANNOT BE

changed, courage to change the things which should be changed, and the wisdom to distinguish the one from the other." When we become centered enough, we have the ability to accept the things we cannot change, and are able to instantly and humbly admit that our willpower and ego are ultimately powerless over most of the realities in our lives.

There are innumerable things we cannot change—the rude salesclerk, the traffic, the flu. Rather than fighting, it is so much simpler to just accept that we aren't in control of these things. Then we can turn our energy toward something more

proactive, such as changing the things we can.

It is so easy to get reactive when we feel like we aren't in control. It happens every day, in a thousand small ways (and sometimes big ones). We spill coffee on ourselves on the way to work, we react. We hit a traffic jam, we react. The boss takes out his or her mood on us, we react. Our kids act up, we react. Again and again we get caught in the endless cycle of stress, reactivity, and blame.

Equanimity is the art of meeting life as it meets you—calmly, without drama or fuss. This is the way out of frustration and into the light. Living in the light, there is a brightness and a creativity very much like that of a child. The light leads us back to our naturalness. But you don't get to the light by fighting or wrestling for control.

An inner revolution is not about taking control. Control has no real healthy place in our lives, and only robs us of our serenity. We think we change things by taking charge, by "grabbing the bull by the horns." But if you think about it, grabbing a bull by the horns would be a crazy thing to do. We change by finding equanimity and learning to relax right in the middle of conflict-filled moments.

Buddha taught that throughout our lives, we should expect to encounter four specific joys and their opposites: pleasure and pain, gain and loss, praise and blame, fame and disrepute. The world conditions us to seek unchanging pleasure, gain, praise, and fame. The problem is that things don't always work out that way. When we experience pain, loss, blame, and disrepute, we take it personally, as if something is deeply wrong with us. Equanimity releases us from unrealistic expectations about what life should be and allows us to stay centered amid the inevitable highs and lows.

Here's a question: Can you see yourself as the same person who maintains composure on a sinking ship, which allows you to help save the lives of others on board? In truth, our equanimity is full of courage and can save lives.

Your focus in Week Three will be to practice equanimity. You will discover that when you want to come out of a pose is the moment you come face-to-face with your psychology. When you hit a threshold—and we all have thresholds—it is an opportunity to see yourself clearly and ask the winds of grace to carry you. Remember, they are always there, willing and ready to carry you if you just raise your sails.

This week, you'll learn why fighting your cravings only leads to more struggle, and how to move through them from a stronger, less reactive space. Your meditation will focus on staying and breathing, no matter what arises, and the excavation questions will illuminate where and when in your life you are most likely to lose your calm, equanimous mind.

Week Three Yoga Practice
45 Minutes

BY NOW, THE SENSE OF FLOW IS PROBABLY WELL INTEGRATED INTO YOUR NERVOUS SYSTEM, SO THE PRACTICE WILL BEGIN TO FEEL MORE AND MORE NATURAL. THIS week, we'll increase our practice time by another fifteen minutes to continue building the healing and purifying heat in your body and take you deeper into the process of transformation.

Beginning Vinyasa

As in the first week of practices, open with the three integration poses: Child's Pose (1), Downward Facing Dog (2), and Ragdoll (3). Then do two rounds of Sun Salutation A and three rounds (one more than last week) of Sun Salutation B. After the third round of Sun Salutation B, go through the steps of Sun Salutation A again until you are in Downward Facing Dog.

Pose 4: Side Plank (Vasisthasana)

From Downward Facing Dog, move forward into High Push-Up position, spin your heels to the right, and take Side Plank (see page 105 for Building Blocks and Alignment).

Connecting Vinyasa

Hold for five breaths, then come back to High Push-Up and go through Vinyasa A until you are in Downward Facing Dog.

From Downward Facing Dog, bring your right leg up to the sky, roll the right hip open, bend the upper knee, and externally open the whole right side of your body. Hold this full-body stretch for five breaths.

Pose 5: Crescent Lunge (Anjaneyasana)

After a few breaths with your upper leg raised, roll open a little more, then step your right foot forward to your right hand for Crescent Lunge (see p. 107 for Building Blocks and Alignment). Hold Crescent Lunge with your hands in a prayerlike position at your heart center for five breaths.

Pose 6: Revolving Crescent Lunge (Parivrtta Alanasana)

Revolving Crescent Lunge is both a heat-building, dynamic pose and a powerful twisting pose that helps transform the health of

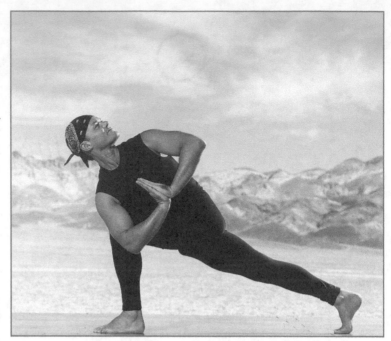

Pose 6: Revolving Crescent Lunge (Parivrtta Alanasana), step 1

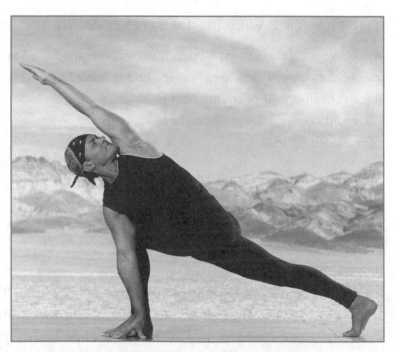

Revolving Crescent Lunge (Parivrtta Alanasana), step 2

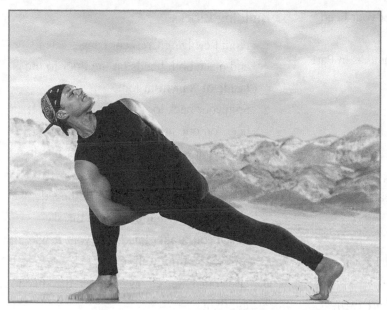

Revolving Crescent Lunge (Parivrtta Alanasana), step 3

2. Keeping your back heel lifted, press through the back leg, lifting the knee toward the ceiling.

3. Stack the front knee over the ankle.

4. Press your palms together to help lengthen your spine and create some space between your torso and your thigh.

5. Roll your torso open; your upper shoulder rolls back, the lower shoulder rolls forward.

6. Look up at the ceiling (or down at the floor if that feels better on your neck).

7. Hold for five breaths.

your internal organs, glands, and circulatory system, as well as the deep muscles and connective tissue of your torso. This pose is done in two parts.

Building Blocks

Part One

1. From Crescent Lunge, exhale and spin your left arm to the outside of the right thigh.

Part Two

8. After five breaths, exhale and straighten your arms, bringing your lower hand to the floor to the outside of your front foot and your upper hand to the sky.

If you want to make this pose more challenging, you can bind your arms as follows:
1. Fold the upper arm down behind your back and wrap your lower arm around your front thigh, bringing it up to meet the upper hand.
2. Make your back leg very strong, press your back foot into the floor, and blossom open through your chest.
3. Work a strong twist, bringing the upper shoulder back and the lower shoulder forward.
4. Lift your torso up off the thigh as much as you can.

9. Reach your upper hand over your head toward the front wall.

10. Everything else stays the same as in Part One.

Alignment

Same as for Crescent Lunge, plus:

- Pull the hip of the front leg back and your chest toward your chin, creating traction through your torso.
- Open your chest wide.
- Pull your wrists back so they are aligned with your elbows (Part One).
- Press through both arms (Part Two).
- Stack your upper hand directly over your shoulder and keep it active (Part Two).
- Drop your shoulder blades down your back.
- Look up past your upper shoulder.

Modification

As in Crescent Lunge, you can drop your back knee to the mat to dilute this movement. In Part Two, you can place your hand to the inside of your foot or use a block.

Pose 7: Extended Side Angle
(Utthita Parsvakonasana)

Extended Side Angle is another full-body pose that opens, stretches, and strengthens the whole body, integrating it as one unit.

Building Blocks

1. From Revolving Crescent Lunge, exhale and place both hands on the floor to the inside of your front foot.

2. Spin your back foot flat (as in Warrior I), heels on one line.

3. Keep your right palm flat on your mat in line with your ankle.

4. Exhale and open your torso to the side, extending your left arm up to the sky.

5. Reach your upper hand over your head toward the front wall.

6. Use your lower elbow to nudge the knee to the right.

7. Gaze at your upper thumbnail.

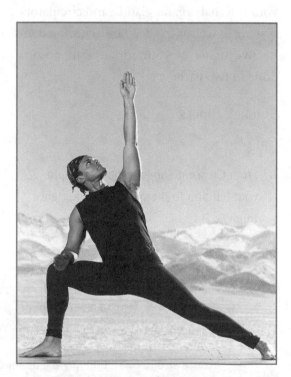

Pose 7: Extended Side Angle (Utthita Parsvakonasana)

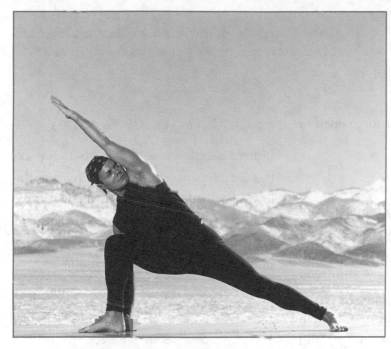

Extended Side Angle (Utthita Parsvakonasana), variation

Alignment

- Keep your heels on one line.
- Press the outer edge of your back foot into the mat.
- Scoop your tailbone down toward the back heel.
- Engage your back thigh, keeping the leg straight and strong.
- Pull your right hip in and under so you can stack your torso on top of your right thigh.
- Keep your heels, hips, and head all on one line.
- Stack your upper shoulder over the lower.
- On the in breath, reach and extend your spine; on the out breath, rinse and spin open a little more.

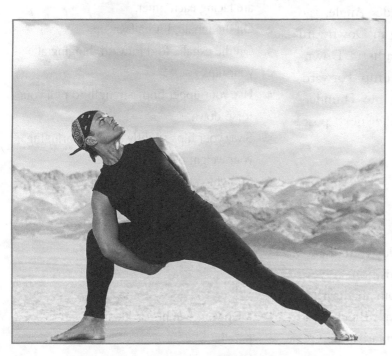

Extended Side Angle (Utthita Parsvakonasana), variation

Modification

If you find that you are leaning forward in order to reach your hand down to the floor, hold on to your ankle or rest your right elbow on top of your right thigh. With this extra height, pull your hip in

To deepen the pose, you can bind your arms by wrapping your upper arm around your back and reaching the other arm down and under your front leg. Interlace your hands and lift your torso up and open.

and under you and roll your torso open to the side wall.

Connecting Vinyasa

After five breaths, release your upper hand down to the mat and step your front foot back, coming into High Push-Up. Go through the steps of Vinyasa A until you are in Downward Facing Dog, then repeat the sequence of Side Plank, Crescent Lunge, Revolving Crescent Lunge, and Extended Side Angle on the left side. After the second Extended Side Angle, go through Vinyasa A, ending in Downward Facing Dog. Take five breaths in Downward Facing Dog, then Jump Forward, bend your knees, and come into Thunderbolt in preparation for the next pose, Prayer Twist.

Pose 8: Prayer Twist (Parivrtta Utkatasana)

From Thunderbolt, exhale your hands down into a prayerlike position at your heart center. Inhale and spin to the right (see page 108 for Building Blocks and Alignment). Hold for five breaths, then release forward into Ragdoll, separating your feet to hip width.

Pose 9: Gorilla Pose (Padhastasana)

Otherwise known as Fingers-to-Toes pose, this is a deep forward bend that releases the lower back and the backs of the legs. Like all forward bends, it restores balance to your biochemistry and allows you to relax into a calm state of concentration.

Building Blocks

1. From Ragdoll, grasp the big toes with the first two fingers of each hand. The palms are facing each other.
2. On the inhale, lift halfway up.
3. On the exhale, fold forward, hinging at your hips.
4. Use your upper body strength to pull your torso down.
5. Sway your hips slightly forward, bringing your weight over your heels.
6. Straighten the knees as much as you can without forcing.
7. Set your eyes to a point directly behind you.

Alignment

- Keep your feet hip width apart and parallel.
- Drop your head.
- Soften your face.

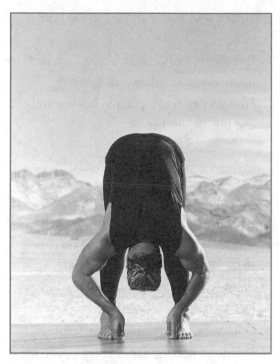

Pose 9: Gorilla Pose (Padhastasana)

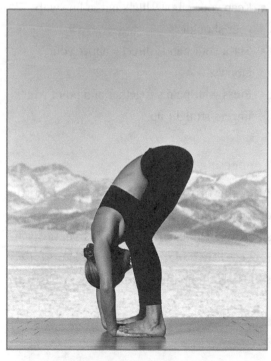

Gorilla Pose (Padhastasana), variation

- Palms face each other.
- Shift your weight into the balls of your feet.
- Sitting bones press up toward the sky.

Modification

You can bend your knees as much as you need to in this pose to feel comfortable.

Connecting Vinyasa

Hold this pose for five breaths, then release your hands and toe/heel your feet back together. Repeat Prayer Twist to the left side, then fold forward again into Gorilla once more, this time placing your hands all the way under your feet, palms up. After the fifth breath, release your hands, toe/heel your feet back together, and slowly come rolling up to standing. End in Samasthiti.

Pose 10: Eagle Pose (Garudasana)

Eagle is a balancing pose, and as with all balancing poses, drishti (your gaze) and breath are key. Balance comes from a calm, centered mind. We set our mind beginning with our eyes, so by fusing your eyes to one point, you bring your mind from distraction to direction. Your breath brings you into the here and now, and facilitates balance by letting you tune out distractions and tune in to your body.

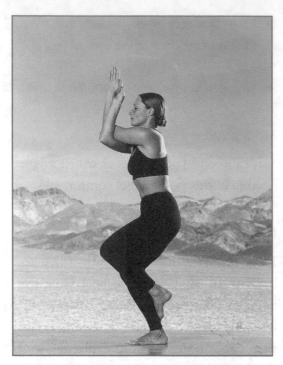

Pose 10: Eagle Pose (Garudasana)

Building Blocks

1. Inhale and sweep your arms up high, alongside your ears.
2. Exhale and wrap your right arm under the left arm like soft rope.
3. Bring your elbows up to shoulder height.
4. Press your palms together and extend your fingers straight up.
5. Bend your knees to a 45-degree angle and sweep your right leg up and over the left.
6. If you can, hook your right foot around the bottom of the left ankle.
7. Square your hips and chest to the front wall.
8. Pull the tops of your shoulders back and down as you lengthen your spine.
9. Fuse your eyes to a point in front of you and breathe for five.

Alignment

- Scoop your tailbone down and under.
- Square your pelvis and hips (imagine you are holding a bowl of water on your pelvic floor and don't want to spill a drop).
- Draw your belly in and up.
- Draw your shoulder blades back.
- Dip down into the standing leg as you lift your torso up.
- Keep your elbows high and in line with your shoulders.
- Stack your hands directly above your elbows.
- Press your palms together and point your fingers straight up.

Connecting Vinyasa

After the fifth exhalation, dip down a little deeper. Inhale and come sweeping up to standing. Repeat the same instructions in reverse for the left side. Take this pose two times on each side, then end in Samasthiti.

To maintain balance, steady your gaze and let your body mold itself around the quiet posture of your mind.

Pose 11: Dancer's Pose (Natarajasana)

Natarajasana translates to "standing bow." In this pose, you want to create a strong tension between your back leg and upper body, as if your legs are the bow and your torso the arrow. This pose teaches you to stabilize your legs and gain an overall greater sense of balance and poise.

Building Blocks

1. From Samasthiti, bring your left arm up to the sky and roll your right hand open so your palm is facing forward.
2. Bend your right knee and bring your right foot up from behind.

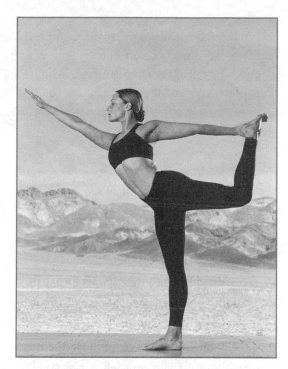

Dancer's Pose (Natarajasana), step 2

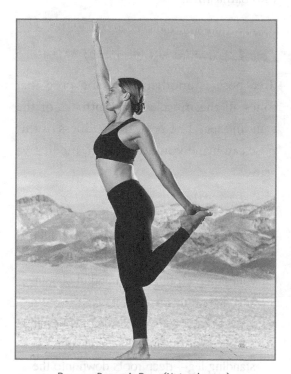

Pose 11: Dancer's Pose (Natarajasana),
step 1, preparation

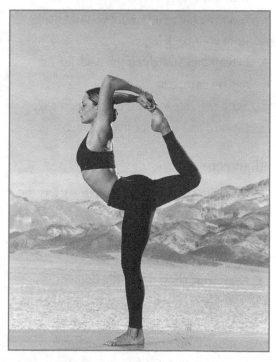

Dancer's Pose (Natarajasana), step 3

For the more advanced variation, begin by using a yoga strap. Bend your right knee and bring your right foot up from behind. Wrap the strap around your right ankle and hold the opposite end of the strap overhead in both hands. Keep your hips squared as you press the upper foot back and the arms up, until you feel a deep stretch in your shoulders and upper back. Keep the standing leg very straight. Eventually, you will be able to work this pose without the strap.

3. Reach your right hand back and grab the inside of your right foot with your thumb pointing up (like a hitchhiker).
4. Bring your knees together.
5. Set your gaze and take a moment to establish your balance and dial into your center line of gravity.
6. Inhale, lift your heart center high, then reach forward with your left arm as you lift your back leg.
7. Come to the point where you can hang from your back leg.
8. Extend and straighten the back leg as much as you can.
9. Set a soft, steady, and determined gaze forward and hold for five breaths.

Alignment

- Maintain strong action in your legs as the "bow."
- Launch your upper body forward, like an arrow.
- Keep your chest up a little higher than your hips.
- Extend your front arm and reach forward through your fingertips.
- Press into the standing leg.

- Spread the toes of the upper foot.
- Fuse your eyes to one point and breathe.

Connecting Vinyasa

After five breaths, release the upper leg down, windmill your arms, and repeat Dancer's Pose on the left side. Repeat the pose once more on each side, then release into Samasthiti.

Pose 12: Tree Pose (Vrksasana)

Tree pose is another balancing pose that tones all the muscles and buttocks of the standing leg. The beautiful stillness of this pose can bring you into a calm, meditative state.

Building Blocks

1. From Samasthiti, lift your right heel high and place the sole of your right foot onto your inner left thigh. Be mindful of your knee here; don't wrench it.
2. Press down through the sole of your left foot, establish your balance on your standing leg—deep roots down into the ground.

3. Drop your right hip down in line with the left.

4. Bring your hands to namaste at your heart center, pressing your palms together. Gaze at your fingertips for five breaths.

5. When you are ready, release your hands, and on the inhalation sweep your hands up above your head, palms facing each other.

6. Interplace your fingers and spin your wrists so your palms face up.

7. Reach up with your entire body.

8. Lift your eyes up.

9. Stand tall and breathe for five.

Alignment

- Maintain a powerful, straight standing leg.
- Keep your hips even (even if that means bringing your raised leg forward a bit).
- Center your hips and pelvis.
- Gently lift and contract your abdominal core.
- Elongate your spine.
- Sustain one central line of energy through your entire body.
- Squeeze your elbows in toward each other.
- Relax your face, neck, and throat.

Connecting Vinyasa

After the second side of Tree Pose, release your arms and legs. Sweep your arms up into Mountain Pose and go through the steps of Vinyasa A, ending in Downward Facing Dog. From Downward Facing Dog, come forward into High Push-Up position. Take one inhalation and one exhala-

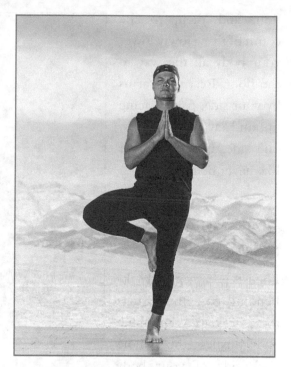

Pose 12: Tree Pose (Vrksasana), step 1

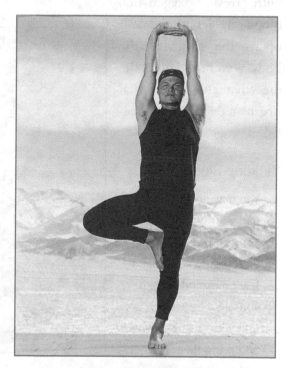

Tree Pose (Vrksasana), step 2

tion, and then, to the count of five, slowly lower your body all the way to the floor. Rest your arms by your side, palms facing up, and lay your head to one side. Love that floor like never before!

Pose 13: Locust (Salabhasana)

Locust is a gentle back-bending pose that brings awareness to your spine and flushes the whole back side of your body with fresh, oxygen-rich blood. It lengthens and opens the front of the body as well, and gives the digestive and other vital organs a deep and powerful massage.

Building Blocks

1. You may need to first pad your hipbones here. You can use a towel or just fold up your mat a few times underneath you.

2. Flip your palms down and bring them in line with your hips, fingers

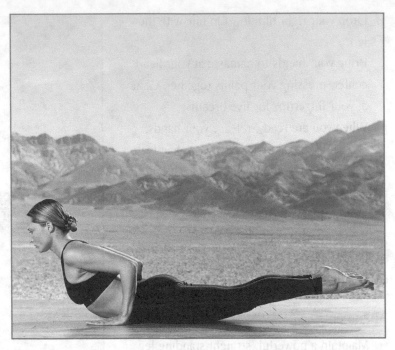

Pose 13: Locust (Salabhasana)

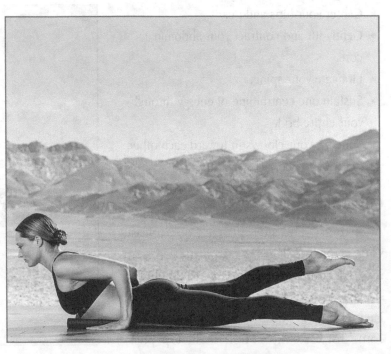

Locust (Salabhasana), modification

facing forward, elbows bent and tucked into your sides.

3. Bring your chin to the floor.
4. Separate your feet to hip width.
5. Inhale, and in one fluid motion lift your chest, ribs, thighs, and feet off the floor.
6. Lower your head so your neck is long and in one line with your spine. The crown of your head should be facing the wall in front of you.

Alignment

- Draw your elbows into your ribs and pull the mat back with your hands.
- Really squeeze your butt and thighs!
- Spin your inner thighs up to the sky.
- Keep your legs straight and active, funneling energy through the balls of your feet.
- Focus on the forward and backward action of your body. On the in breath, extend your chest forward; on the out breath, extend your legs back and up, as though someone were behind you pulling them out of your hip sockets.
- Drop your shoulder blades down toward your hips.

Modification

If this bothers your lower back, you can bring one leg up at a time. Do the right leg, then the left.

Connecting Vinyasa

After five breaths, relax down and rest one cheek on your mat. Repeat the pose a second time, resting on the other cheek when you are done.

Pose 14: Bow Pose (Dhanurasana)

Bow Pose continues the stimulating effects of backbends and conditions the back side of the body. It is also an amazing chest opener and a profound release for the fronts of the shoulders, hips, and thighs.

Building Blocks

1. From the resting position after Locust, bring your chin back to the floor.
2. Bend your knees and bring them to hip width.

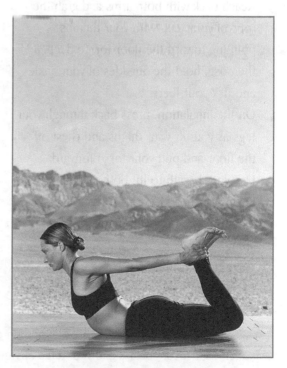

Pose 14: Bow Pose (Dhanurasana)

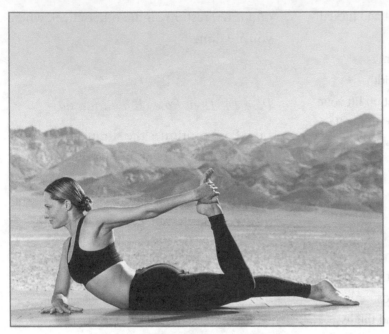

Bow Pose (Dhanurasama), modification

Alignment

- Activate your feet and spread your toes.
- Spiral your inner thighs to the ceiling.
- Maintain very strong legs as the anchor from which your torso is suspended.
- Drop your head forward to let the neck muscles stretch.
- Soften your face.

Modification

As with Locust, if this hurts your lower back, bring one leg up at time.

Connecting Vinyasa

After five breaths, release your arms and legs and lower back down to the floor, bringing your cheek to one side. Take two deep breaths, and then bring your hands to the floor, palms facing down, hands by your ribs. Press down and come into Upward Dog for three long breaths. Inhale, lift your heart higher and then exhale and roll over your toes to Downward Dog.

From there, take the following three back-bending poses, as you did in Week Two:

3. Reach back with both arms and grab the tops of your feet, with your thumbs pointing toward the floor (or, to deepen the pose, hold the outsides of your ankles and flex your feet).
4. On the inhalation, press back through your legs as you lift your thighs and chest off the floor and pull your torso forward.
5. Use your breath to lift both ends up.
6. Drop your head forward so your neck is in a neutral position with the rest of your spine.
7. Gaze down to the floor.
8. Breathe through any tension.

The tighter the bow, the more spring you get from the arrow. Use the power of your legs to launch your chest upward and your torso forward.

Pose 15: Camel Pose

(page 109)

Take the pose two times, ending in Downward Facing Dog. Come to your hands and knees, cross the feet and roll over your feet, coming onto your back on your mat.

Pose 16: Bridge Pose

(page 111)

After taking the pose, lower back to your mat. Either repeat Bridge Pose a second time, or move to wheel.

Pose 17: Wheel

(page 112)

Take Wheel two times, then lower back to your mat. Rest with your legs extended out for three to five breaths.

Pose 18: Scissor Legs and 60/30 Lift

This two-part pose tones and strengthens the entire abdominal wall. Unlike

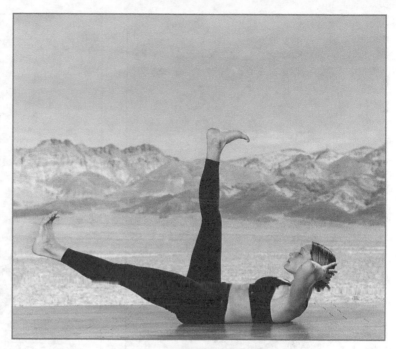

Pose 18: Scissor Legs

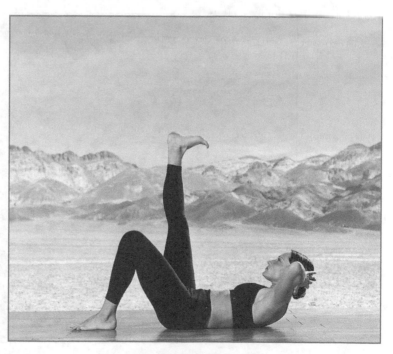

Scissor Legs Modification

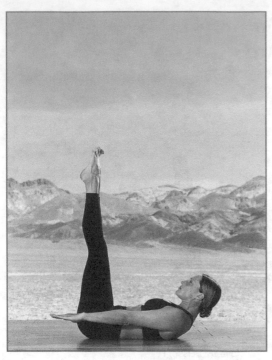

60/30 Lift (1)

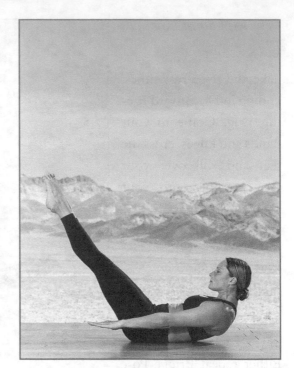

60/30 Lift (2)

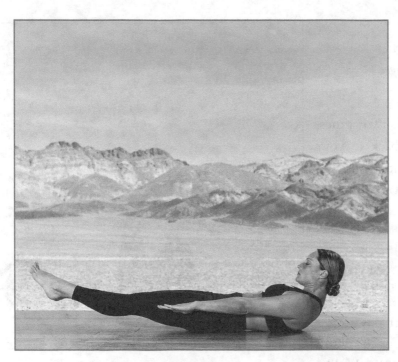

60/30 Lift (3)

regular fitness crunches, these movements are global body movements: Besides toning and strengthening your abs, they integrate and coordinate the upper, lower, and midbody in such a way that provide real-life flexible strength to infuse even your regular daily movements with ease and grace.

Building Blocks

Part One

1. From the resting position after Wheel, bring your knees into your chest and give them a squeeze.
2. Cradle your head with your hands and extend your legs straight up to the sky.
3. Lower your right leg down to one foot above the floor.
4. Flex your feet and press through both of your legs to keep them strong.
5. Lift your head and shoulders off the floor.
6. Inhale, then exhale and contract your belly in toward the floor as you pulse your torso up for ten counts.
7. Exhale as you lift up and contract your abdominal wall; match your breath to your movements.

8. After ten pulses, reverse your legs for another count often.

Part Two

9. After the count of ten, bring both legs up and your arms out parallel to the floor (or you can keep cradling your head if your neck needs support).
10. Keep your shoulder blades off the floor.
11. Lower your legs down 30 degrees and hold for five breaths.
12. Lower your legs down another 30 degrees and hold for five breaths.
13. Lower your legs until your heels are two inches off the floor and hold for five breaths.
14. Release your heels down to the floor and lie on your back in position for the following pose, Supta Baddha Konasana.

Modification

If you feel strain in your lower back, bend one knee and place the sole of that foot into the floor.

When I used to teach in Paris and I would ask if the students wanted to do any abdominal work, the answer was always No. When I ask students in America, the answer is always a resounding Yes. We are obsessed with the appearance of sleek abs, yet the real benefit of these movements is the deeper seat of power and inner strength you gain that stabilizes every move you make. Everything you do becomes much easier and lighter when you operate from a strong and stable core. The nice by-product, of course, is that you can end up with really toned and sculpted abs.

Pose 19: *Supta Baddha Konasana*

This is a neutralizing pose that soothes the nervous system, releases the lower back as well as the hips, and stretches the inner thigh muscles. As you drop into the floor and surrender to this pose, all your internal organs and body systems are rebalanced and revitalized.

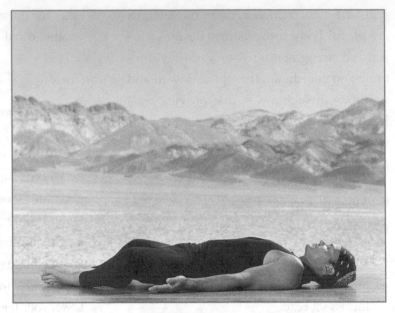

Pose 19: Supta Baddha Konasana

Building Blocks

1. From the horizontal prone position, bend your knees and bring the soles of your feet together, letting your legs and knees splay open to the sides.
2. Lay your arms by your sides with your palms facing up (or, if you prefer, rest your hands on your belly).
3. Close your eyes.

Alignment

- Your feet should be about one or two feet away from your groin.
- Scoop your tailbone under, drawing the front of your pelvis up toward your ribs.
- Let the valley of your pelvis sink into the earth.
- Drop your belly.
- Drop your brain.
- Take deep rest.

Connecting Vinyasa

When you are ready, bring your knees into your chest and rock-and-roll five times up and back, ending in a seated position with your knees bent and the soles of your feet flat on the floor.

Pose 20: *Boat Pose (Navasana)*

From the seated position, take Boat Pose once, following it with one cross-and-lift action (see p. 114 for Building Blocks and Alignment). Finish back in the seated position with the soles of your feet on the floor.

Pose 21: Rock the Baby
(Vinyaspadmasana)

This pose, like all the hip openers, is important because it frees up the body to sit comfortably, both in meditation and in everyday life. It increases the range of motion in the hip joints, releasing tightness and increasing circulation.

Building Blocks

1. Place the right foot in the crook of the left elbow.
2. Bring the right arm around the knee and clasp your hands, cradling the leg in your arms.

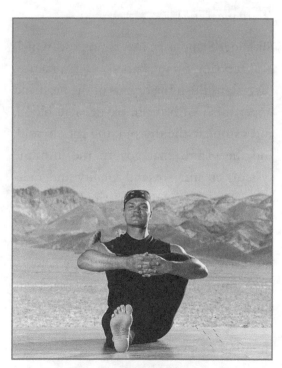

Pose 21: Rock the Baby (Vinyaspadmasana)

3. Flex the right heel and lift the right foot up until the right shinbone is horizontal, level with the floor.
4. Gently pull the leg in toward your chest.
5. Gaze forward and hold for five breaths.

Alignment

- Bring your leg toward your chest and your chest toward your leg.
- Lift and straighten your spine.
- Broaden your chest.
- Relax your shoulders.

Pose 22: Bent Leg Seated Twist
(Marichyasana)

This pose is an overall counterbalance that creates a deep twist for your entire spine and frees up your lower back.

Building Blocks

1. From Rock the Baby, release your right leg and place the sole of your right foot flat on the floor to the outside of your left hip.
2. Tuck your left foot underneath your right butt cheek.
3. Place your right hand directly behind you as a support.
4. Reach your left arm up, bend the elbow, and place the elbow to the outside of the right knee.
5. Take a deep breath in, lengthen your spine.
6. Exhale and twist your torso open.

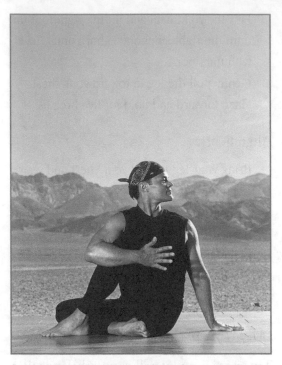

Pose 22: Bent Leg Seated Twist (Marichyasana)

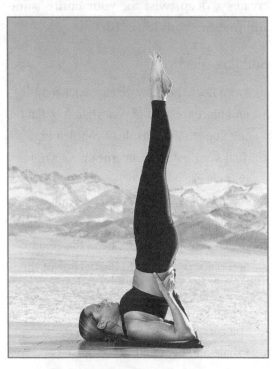

Pose 23: Shoulder Stand (Sarvangasana)

Alignment

- Press down into your right hand to lengthen your spine.
- Leverage your left elbow against your right knee to help you twist your torso open.

Connecting Vinyasa

After five breaths in Seated Twist, come back to center and release your legs back to the seated position. Repeat the sequence of Rock the Baby and Bent Leg Seated Twist on the other side, ending in the seated position.

Pose 23: Shoulder Stand (Sarvangasana)

Shoulder Stand is an inversion pose, which is a very important part of yoga practice. Inversions flush the organs in the head and upper torso with fresh, oxygenated blood, and stimulate the thyroid, the parathyroid, and the glands that govern the immune system, creating overall vitality and radiance. They also drain the fluids from the legs and hips to create suppleness in the lower body. Reversing the flow of gravity moves lymph, which is the body's "sewage," through your system, so metabolic waste can be released.

Building Blocks

1. From the seated position, roll onto your back so you are flat on your mat.

2. Contract your abdominal muscles and, on the exhalation, lift your legs up to the sky, placing your hands facing down into the mat, under your tail.
3. Press down in your hands as you lift your hips up high, rolling onto the backs of your shoulders.
4. Bring your hands to your lower back and walk your elbows and shoulder blades in toward each other.
5. Press up through the soles of your feet, using your hands to support your hips and lift them higher.
6. Soften your eyes and set them on the tip of your nose or on your toes.
7. Hold for ten breaths.

Alignment

- Relax your neck and throat.
- It is *very important* that you look straight up, never to the right or left, to protect your neck.
- Press your shoulders and elbows down into your mat.
- Walk your elbows in towards each other.
- Spiral your inner thighs in toward each other.
- Press through the balls of the feet, inner anklebones touching.

Modification

If you have lower back or neck problems, you might want to modify by stopping at step 2 of Building Blocks. Leave your hips and lower back on the floor with your legs straight up to the sky. Hold here for the full ten breaths.

Connecting Vinyasa

After ten breaths, lower your knees slowly into your chest and come rolling down slowly, vertebra by vertebra. Extend your legs out straight in preparation for the next pose, Fish Pose.

Pose 24: Fish Pose (Matsyasana)

Fish Pose is a wonderful counterbalancing pose that releases the muscles in the back and opens the throat, chest, and entire front side of the torso, bringing the body back into balance.

Building Blocks

1. Place your hands under your sitting muscles, palms facing down.
2. Lean back until your forearms are down on the floor.

The image you want to hold in your mind of this pose is of a candle flame in a quiet room: still and straight. The fluctuations of the mind show up in the body, so calm your mind and still your flame.

3. Walk your elbows and forearms in toward each other, then shimmy your shoulder blades in toward each other.

4. On the inhalation, raise your heart muscle high and arch your back, then lower your head back and slide back until the crown is resting on the floor or to whatever point where you stop.

5. Create a big, beautiful bend in your upper back, opening your throat and heart to the heavens.

6. Gaze to a point on the wall behind you and breathe deeply for five inhalations and exhalations.

Alignment

- Point and activate your toes.
- Keep your feet together, inner anklebones touching.
- Root your forearms down into the floor.
- Engage your thighs.
- Root the hips down and lift your heart muscle high.

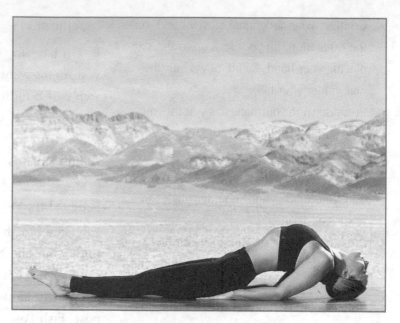

Pose 24: Fish Pose (Matsyasana)

Connecting Vinyasa

After five breaths, inhale, lift your head up, tuck your chin, slowly release your arms, and lower back down into the horizontal resting position.

Pose 25: Supine Leg Raise, Front (Supta Urdhva Padangustasana)

This pose teaches active rest. As you soothe and calm your nervous system, you are also allowing a deep release in the hamstrings, lower back, and hips.

Fish Pose stimulates and opens the throat and heart areas, which energetically store our self-expression and intuition. You may experience some powerful release in this pose in the shape of inspiration or deep understanding. Whatever truths arise, remember that it is these very truths that can ultimately set you free.

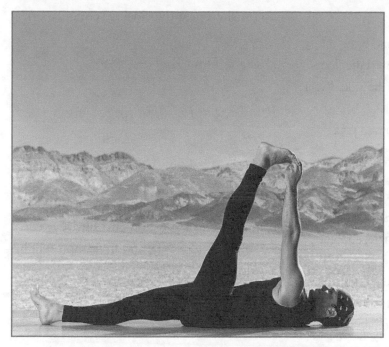

Pose 25: Supine Leg Raise, Front (Supta Urdhva Padangustasana)

Building Blocks

1. Lying on your back with both legs straight and strong, raise the right leg and grasp the big toe with the first two fingers of the right hand.
2. Bring your left hand onto your left thigh.
3. Straighten the raised leg as much as possible without rounding your back.
4. Gaze up at your raised foot and breathe for five.

Alignment

- Keep both feet active.
- Keep your abdomen long, hollow, and empty.
- Broaden your chest.
- Soften your face.

Pose 26: Supine Leg Raise, Side

This pose is deeply restful for the whole body. It opens the hips and stretches the adductors, groin, and neck.

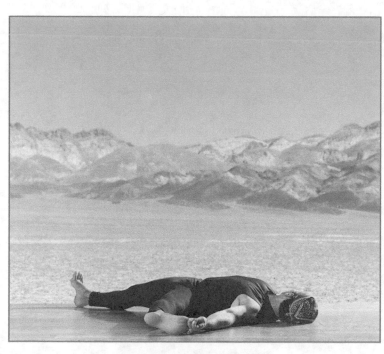

Pose 26: Supine Leg Raise, Side

Building Blocks

1. From Supine Leg Raise, Front, bring the right leg out to the side toward the floor.
2. Extend your left arm out to the side, like a wing.
3. Turn your head and gaze toward your extended left arm.

Alignment

- Flatten your shoulder blades into the floor.
- Your arms should form a single, straight line.
- Keep your sacrum flat into the floor.
- Take the leg only as far as it will go without tipping your body to one side.

To finish, repeat the closing sequence of:

Pose 27: Dead Bug (page 89)

Pose 28: Supine Twist (page 116)

Pose 29: Savasana (page 90)

End by rolling over onto your right side, bringing your hands to your third-eye center, breathing deeply, and inviting the light as you say, "Namaste."

For a quick reference to this week's poses, see page 237.

Week Three Balancing Diet

In general, mankind, since the improvement of cookery,
eats twice as much as nature requires.

—BENJAMIN FRANKLIN

THE THEME OF WEEK THREE IS EQUANIMITY, AND THERE IS NO PLACE WHERE REACTIVITY SHOWS UP FASTER THAN IN OUR DIETS. WE GET STRESSED AND WE GRAB FOR

something to eat, usually something sweet. We feel anxious and we immediately reach for "comfort foods." We feel lonely, depressed, and unworthy, and without missing a beat, we have our hands in a bag of chips or are steering our cars up to the drive-in window at the nearest fast-food restaurant.

A good appetite is considered healthy, but too much of an appetite is a whole other thing. A lot of people base their appetite not on true physical hunger, but on a deeper, gnawing spiritual emptiness. They overeat not because they are excessively hungry, but because they mindlessly

shovel food into their mouths the minute an uncomfortable truth or feeling arises, as a way to hide. The idea of staying with the hurricane within is just too unbearable to them, and they go on autopilot to make sure they stay very firmly within the boundaries of their comfort zones. But as we know, we *must* step out of our comfort zones if we want to grow. We have to pass through what is messy and sometimes painful if we are to get to the bliss on the other side.

One of the best ways to understand the underlying nature of our appetite is by looking at what we crave. We tend to crave different things at different times—sometimes we want something salty, other times we just want *a lot* of food, but the craving for something sweet is the most common in our culture. The root of the word *nutrition* stems from the Sanskrit word *snauti,* which means "suckle." In many ways, when we crave something sweet, we want to satisfy ourselves, comfort ourselves, fill ourselves up. We are trying to get that feeling of being at our mother's bosom. Psychologists say that most issues involving food revolve around mothers' love, or lack thereof.

Sugar has not always been so readily available to us as it is today, with candy and other sweets being thrown at us at every turn. When ancient Egyptian soldiers were severely injured in battle, they were treated with a little sugar dripped into their mouths. Imagine sugar being so precious that it had the power to help a badly injured man to his feet! We've come a long way since then, with white sugar never more than arm's reach away. It has become commonplace; we have the ability to buy it cheaply and everywhere. We consume it whenever life isn't going our way, because, as those soldiers discovered hundreds of centuries ago, it feels good.

Ancient Chinese medicine practitioners realized long ago that when the body reacts adversely to life, it craves sweets. In those moments of resistance, when you

Now more than ever, science is proving that our bodies need healthy, clean, and vibrant nourishment; otherwise disease sets in. This validates what many of us understand on an intuitive level. So why do we intelligent humans still consume lifeless fast-food cheeseburgers and fries and pour soda down our throats and those of our children? The answer is easy. We are living out our legacy of distraction. It is easier to distract ourselves and go along with the status quo than to feel the discomfort of growth and change.

We may not realize it, but we are literally involved in biological warfare with ourselves. We use what I call "biological grenades"—drugs, sex, sugar, food—to continually alter our chemistry in order to avoid coming to peace with ourselves. We shift our moods to create a wall of separation between reality and ourselves, then blame these biological grenades as the problem.

We believe that these distractions have their own power and energy, but really, it is our attachment to them that gives them their fuel. Our distractions are powered by our own minds, by the need to lie to ourselves about ourselves. Ultimately, we can break our patterns only by leaning into them and acknowledging them fully, not by drowning them out or trying to cover them up with yet another biological grenade.

What a lot of us don't realize is that the sweet taste doesn't show up only in the form of sugar. There is a broad range of sweet tastes, extending from fruits to vegetables all the way to dairy products and good-quality meats. We are just so used to the high-octane hit of sweetness we get from candy, cookies, and so on that we have lost our ability to feel satisfied by the less obvious, more subtle sensations of sweet gratification.

The less reactive you become and the more high-quality, fresh foods you eat on a regular basis, the less of a sweet "hit" you will need to get that feeling of being satisfied.

tense up rather than relax with what is, you fail to meet life as it meets you, and you create a chemical reaction in your body that demands to be soothed. It works like this: Let's say you are in a rush, and as you turn the corner in your car, you encounter a massive traffic jam. The instant you lose your equanimous mind and get reactive, upset, and/or angry, you cease to go with the flow of life, and you trigger that chemical reaction in your body. When you need soothing, you crave sweets. Twenty minutes later, you may have forgotten all about the traffic, but your body hasn't. The craving is hardly ever really about the situation; rather, it's about the feeling that the situation is creating in you.

Week Three Diet To-Do

During this week, as you continue to choose vibrant, fresh, whole foods to balance your body, think about what sweetness means to you. When do you usually crave the taste? Do you consider things such as candy, cookies, and other sweets necessities? If so, why do you think that is? Do you resist what comes up in life, and fail to meet it as it meets you?

Throughout the week, when you have a craving to run for the cookie jar or to fill yourself up with something sweet, take a moment to be still, breathe, and seek the truth of what is really going on. Interrupt your habitual pattern and ask yourself hon-

Probably one of the most important reminders about appetite is to eat until you are two-thirds full. There is about a fifteen-to-twenty-minute lag between eating and feeling satiated; it takes roughly this long for the message that you are full to get from your stomach to your brain. If you envision your stomach as a furnace or cauldron, you'll realize that if you pack it too tightly, things will not burn efficiently. If you leave space for air, the fire of your digestive process will work its magic, giving you energy and vitality, rather than slowing you down.

A craving for salt is not the same as one for sweetness. We crave sweets for energy and comfort, but we crave salt for minerals and grounding. If you crave salt, you will want to incorporate more mineral-rich foods such as fish, seaweed, and green leafy vegetables into your diet to bring you into balance.

estly what is causing it. Did you just get some bad news? Do you want to numb out? Are you trying to hide something? More often than not, if we are really truthful with ourselves, we will see that the overeating or the craving isn't the problem; rather, it's the issue below the surface that this craving is masking.

As I've said, the practices in this book are a study in the art of staying. Even if you think you might die if you don't have a chocolate bar, stay and breathe. Even if it feels terrifying to sit with the truths that are coming up, stay and breathe anyway. The more you can ride out the storms within, the clearer the horizon will be.

Week Three Equanimity Meditation

15 minutes

MEDITATION IS A POWERFUL TOOL FOR NOTICING AND LETTING GO OF OUR HABITUAL RE-SPONSES. IN OUR DAILY LIVES, THE GREATEST CHALLENGE TO OUR equanimity is our reactivity—the automatic response of resistance and resentment we have when we encounter anything that is uncomfortable. A calm, equanimous mind does not react to circumstances or sensations around it and can turn the poison of distraction and aversion into nectar for growth.

Set your intention to sit with strong determination. Resolve not to quit before the fifteen minutes are up. Simply and gently notice your reluctance to meditate, your desire to stop or get up and walk out of the room. Notice the urge to fidget, to move your posture, to scratch an itch, resolve not to give in to these feelings. When these restless behaviors arise, rather than just acting on them and your need to escape, see if you can just notice their pull on you. Stay present, stay conscious, and most of all, just *stay*. This is the practice of developing equanimity.

Do this practice for fifteen minutes each morning and fifteen minutes each evening this week.

Equanimity Excavation Questions

1. How much do I believe that the winds of grace support me, and how does this play out in my everyday life?

2. In what areas of my life can I have less reaction and more divine interpretation? For instance, in my relationships, when things get stressful at work, when I'm stuck in traffic, when I make a mistake, and so on.

3. How can I enhance the quality of my life through a shift in my attitude? How would situations feel different if I practiced nonreactivity, rather than launching into an automatic response?

4. What things are most likely to trigger reactivity in me?

5. What can I do in those moments of reactivity to respond better? Take a walk? Take A breath? Remind myself that every circumstance is an opportunity to practice equanimity?

Week Four: Restoration

THE TIME TO RELAX IS WHEN YOU DON'T HAVE THE TIME FOR IT. MOST OF US ARE ALWAYS PUSHING OURSELVES TO THE LIMIT, CONVINCING OURSELVES THAT WE WILL

be content only when we are working our to-do list. We can't seem to find time for ourselves or for others as we rush through life. So often we say to ourselves, "I wish I had the time to do this" or "There isn't enough time."

As we remove the rocks that block our wisdom and light, we find that we are able to set more and more time aside for the things that restore us: time spent in nature, solitude, meditation, intimacy, having heart-to-heart conversations that heal. These moments spent in restoring ourselves are signposts of our progress in health.

Leonardo da Vinci was one of the most creative figures in history. He accomplished so much in his lifetime as a master painter, inventor, and thinker. It would appear as though the guy was a type A who never took time for anything but work. However, it was he who gave this piece of sage advice, which I am sure came out of his own need to find harmony and balance: "Every now and then go away, have a little relaxation, for when you come back to your work your judgment will be surer. . . . [G]o some distance away, because the work appears smaller and more of it can be taken in at a glance, and a lack of harmony or proportion is more readily seen."

As someone who keeps a very full schedule as a father, teacher, writer, and speaker, I have learned the great power of taking time out to create sanctuary. I have had to learn to pace myself, to learn when to retreat and escape from the daily grind and take some time to clear my head, rest my body, and restore my soul. When I find myself being consumed—which can happen pretty quickly—it is very important that I step back, gain some space, and let my closeness to the things of my life dissolve. This distance clears my head and gives me renewed vision and energy, which then boost my productivity and creativity and expand my worldview. Things that seemed so big now appear much smaller and more manageable. I always gain new insights when I let go of my work and life for a period of time.

When students come to my weeklong bootcamps, it is a chance to put the noise and business of their lives on hold for seven days and take a restorative retreat. I recognize that not everyone can leave their lives entirely for seven days, but to the best of your ability, your focus this week will be on your own personal restoration. As often as you can during the next seven days, carve out time and space to restore yourself in mind, body, and spirit.

This is the week of the three-day fruit fast, in which you will fully cleanse your body. The cleanse will leave you lighter,

cleaner, and infused with more energy. During the days you are detoxing, I encourage you to take everything in your life a little bit easier. Take time in solitude, to rest or to do things that restore you in small ways.

Throughout the cleanse, you will continue your daily meditation practice, increasing it to twenty minutes. If you want to experiment, you can break the time up into three or four smaller chunks throughout the day. Meditating this way has proven to be a salvation for me. If I have had an emotionally challenging or upsetting experience and I feel that my judgment is off or that resentment has reared its ugly head, I know to remove myself and sit quietly in order to restore myself to sanity.

Your daily yoga practice will increase to sixty minutes this week. Some students worry at first that they will not be able to practice yoga while cleansing, but in fact, as soon as we remove the heavy burden of digestion from our bodies, we are able to do so much more. In fact—and this is optional—you may want to try doing another short practice sometime in the afternoon, in addition to your morning routine (you can either use the practice in Week One or just do whatever asanas feel intuitively right to you). Very often the afternoon is a regrouping for me. I'll take twenty minutes or so of asanas, just to center myself in my body and move or shift the energy.

Throughout this week, remember to stay in the moment and relax in all of your activities. Put aside your focus on outcomes and meeting expectations for right now. If you get stuck in tension and toxic behaviors, rather than launching into old patterns, be like Moses at the Red Sea: Realize you are in over your head and unconditionally surrender everything over to God.

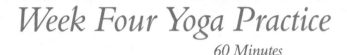

Week Four Yoga Practice
60 Minutes

THIS IS THE WEEK OF YOUR CLEANSE, WHICH WILL RESTORE YOUR BODY AND SPIRIT ON A WHOLE OTHER LEVEL. LET GO OF ANY RESISTANCE YOU HAVE IN YOUR

practice this week, and you'll see that you can do more than you think you can. Drop your brain, drop your expectations, and just let go and flow.

Beginning Vinyasa

As in the first week of practice, open with the three integration poses: Child's Pose (1), Downward Facing Dog (2), and Ragdoll (3). Then do three (one more than last week) rounds of Sun Salutation A and three rounds of Sun Salutation B, ending in Downward Facing Dog.

Pose 4: Side Plank (Vasisthasana)

From Downward Facing Dog, move forward into High Push-Up, spin your heels to the right, and take Side Plank (see p. 105 for Building Blocks and Alignment). Hold for five breaths.

Connecting Vinyasa

Come back to High Push-Up and go through vinyasa A again, ending in Downward Facing Dog. From Downward Facing Dog, bring your right leg up to the sky, bend the upper knee, and externally rotate the whole front right side of your body open. Hold this full-body stretch for five breaths.

Pose 5: Crescent Lunge
(Anjaneyasana)

Square your hips and lunge your raised leg forward to your hands, sweeping up on the inhale into Crescent Lunge (see p. 107 for Building Blocks and Alignment). On the exhale, bring your hands to namaste at your heart center. Hold here for five breaths.

Pose 6: Revolving Crescent Lunge
(Parivrtta Alanasana)

Exhale and spin your left arm to the outside of your right thigh, coming into Revolving Crescent Lunge (see p. 126 for Building Blocks and Alignment). Hold for five breaths.

Connecting Vinyasa

After five breaths, release your hands down to the mat on either side of your front foot and step back into High Push-Up. Go through the steps of vinyasa A until you are in Downward Facing Dog, then repeat the sequence of Side Plank, Crescent Lunge, and Revolving Crescent Lunge on the left side. After the second Extended Side Angle, go through vinyasa A, ending in Downward Facing Dog.

Pose 7: Thunderbolt (Utkatasana)

Take five breaths in Downward Facing Dog and then jump or walk forward to your hands. Lift halfway up and then fold forward into Standing Forward Bend. Bend your knees, dip your hips, and sweep your arms up, coming into Thunderbolt (see p. 76 for Building Blocks and Alignment). Hold here for five breaths.

Pose 8: Prayer Twist
(Parivrtta Utkatasana)

From Thunderbolt, bring your hands down to your heart center, inhale, and spin the left elbow past the right thigh, coming into Prayer Twist (see page 108 for Building Blocks and Alignment).

Connecting Vinyasa

After five breaths, release forward into Ragdoll. Toe/heel your feet to hip width in preparation for Gorilla Pose.

Put your thoughts, effort, and resistance aside and let the universe work on your behalf. If you are relaxing, you are receiving. Even if it's hard, relax anyway.

Pose 9: Gorilla Pose (Padhastasana)

Hook the first two fingers of each hand around the big toes. Inhale and lift halfway up, then exhale and fold forward, coming into Gorilla Pose (see p. 130 for Building Blocks and Alignment). Hold for five breaths.

Connecting Vinyasa

After the fifth breath, release your hands and toe/heel your feet back together. Repeat Prayer Twist to the left side, then fold forward again into Gorilla, this time taking the variation of placing your hands all the way under your feet, palms up. After the fifth breath, release your hands, toe/heel your feet back together, and slowly come rolling up to standing. Sweep your arms up high to the sky, coming into Mountain Pose.

Pose 10: Eagle Pose (Garudasana)

From Mountain Pose, sweep up into Eagle Pose (p. 131), two times on each side. End in Samasthiti.

Pose 11: Dancer's Pose (Natarajasana)

From Samasthiti, bring your left arm up and bend your right knee, grabbing the inside of your right foot. Exhale and launch forward, coming into Dancer's Pose (p.

133). Hold for five breaths, remembering to fuse your eyes to one point.

Connecting Vinyasa

After five breaths, release the upper leg down and repeat Dancer's Pose on the left side. Repeat the pose once more on each side, then release into Samasthiti.

Pose 12: Tree Pose (Vrksasana)

From the standing position, take Tree Pose (p. 134), one time on each leg. Hold for five breaths.

Connecting Vinyasa

After the last breath on the second side of Tree Pose, release your arms and leg. Go through vinyasa B, ending in Warrior I on the right side.

Pose 13: Triangle (Trikonasana)

From Warrior I, take Warrior II. Straighten your right knee on track and reach your right arm forward, moving into Triangle Pose (see p. 104).

Connecting Vinyasa

After the fifth exhalation, inhale and let your raised arm pull you up to standing. Close your front foot so both feet are parallel. This puts you in position for the next pose, Standing Straddle Bend C.

Pose 14: Standing Straddle Bend C (Prasarita C)

This deep hamstring and calf stretch is also an inversion, which allows for deep release as it quiets and soothes the nervous system. The arm position also provides a wonderful stretch for the front of your shoulders.

Building Blocks

1. Facing the side wall, turn your toes in a bit so your feet are slightly pigeontoed.
2. Interlace your hands behind your back with your arms straight.

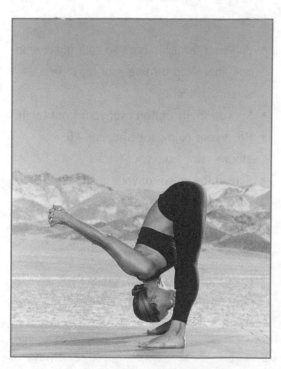

Pose 14: Standing Straddle Bend C (Prasarita C)

3. On the next inhalation, lift your chest and chin upward, bringing a slight arch to your back.
4. On the exhalation, hinge forward from your hips, wrapping your arms over your head toward the floor in front of you.

Alignment

- Lift your inner anklebones and press into the outer edges of your feet.
- Sway your hips forward so they are in line with your heels.
- Lift your sitting bones and spread them away from each other.
- Keep your arms active
- Keep your eyes and face soft and relaxed.

Connecting Vinyasa

After five breaths, use your abdominal muscles to pull you back up to standing.

Pose 15: Pyramid Pose (Parsvottanasana)

This is an intense stretch that gets way down deep into the hamstrings.

Building Blocks

1. From the standing position after Standing Straddle Bend, open your right foot to face the front of the room.
2. Bring your hands to your hips.

3. Square your hips and your torso to the front of the room. You may need to step your back foot in a little bit to do this.

4. On the inhalation, root down into your legs and lift your chin and chest up, slightly arching your back.

5. On the exhalation, hinge forward over your front leg.

6. Release your hands to the floor.

7. Walk your hands as far back as you can with your fingers facing the back wall, palms flat, elbows straight.

8. Gaze to the big toe of your back foot.

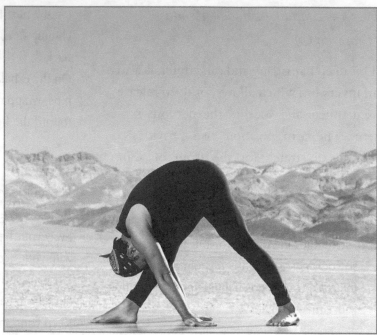

Pose 15: Pyramid Pose (Parsvottanasana)

Alignment

- Maintain a strong, straight back leg.
- Square your hips and chest to the front of the room.
- Press the front thigh and sitting bones back.

- Pull your front hip back so your hips are in one line. Keep turning your hips like a steering wheel.
- Set your belly button over your front thigh.
- Press your palms together and lift your elbows away from your back.
- Extend the crown of your head down toward your front foot.
- Relax your head, neck, and face.

If you get dizzy in this pose, know that it is natural and that it will pass. It is just all the stuck and toxic energy coming up for release. Welcome it, because the sooner it comes up and out, the sooner you will be free of it. If you do get dizzy, DO NOT close your eyes; this will only make it worse. Keep your eyes open, stay alert, and remember to breathe. If you need to, you can always come down into Child's Pose.

Modification

You can bend the front knee if you need to, but eventually the leg should be straight.

Connecting Vinyasa

After five breaths, change your hand position so your fingers are facing forward and step back into High Push-Up. Go through vinyasa A, ending in Downward Facing Dog. Repeat the sequence of Triangle and Pyramid Pose with your left leg forward. After the second repetition, go through vinyasa A once again, ending in Downward Facing Dog. From Downward Facing Dog, move forward to High Push-Up and, to the count of five, slowly lower the front of your body down to the mat.

From there, take the following backbending sequence, as you did in Week Three:

Pose 16: Locust Pose (page 136)

Take Locust Pose two times. End with your cheek to one side on your mat.

Pose 17: Bow Pose (page 137)

Take Bow Pose two times. End with your cheek to one side on your mat.

Pose 18: Camel Pose (page 109)

Take Bow Pose two times, resting in Downward Facing Dog in between. End in Downward Facing Dog. Come onto your hands and knees, cross your feet, roll over your heels, and get into position for Bridge.

Pose 19: Bridge Pose (page 111)

Take Bridge Pose one time, then lower back to your mat. Either repeat Bridge three more times for a total of four, or take just one Bridge and then move to the next pose, Wheel.

Pose 20: Wheel (page 112)

Take Wheel three times, lowering down to your mat in between for two breaths. Rest with your legs extended out for three to five breaths.

Pose 21: Dead Bug
(Urdhva Mukha Upavista Konasana)

Bring your knees up to your chest, grab the inner edges of your feet, and take Dead Bug Pose (p. 89) for five breaths.

Connecting Vinyasa

After five breaths, release your feet.

Then take the following abdominal sequence.

Pose 22: *Scissor Legs and 60/30 Lift*

Do one set of scissor legs (pulsing up for ten on each leg), one 60/30 lift. Then move to Abdominal Twists.

Pose 23: *Abdominal Twists*

This movement integrates your whole body to strengthen and tone the core muscles down deep, especially the obliques, which are the stabilizing muscles for the lower back.

Building Blocks

1. Squeeze your knees into your chest and cradle your head.
2. Stack your knees over your hips and bring your elbows up to touch your knees, hold.
3. Then extend your right leg and twist your torso over to the left side, hold for 5 breaths.
4. Come to center and touch your elbows to your knees.

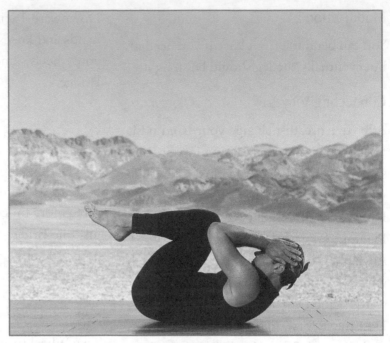

Abdominal Twists (step 1)

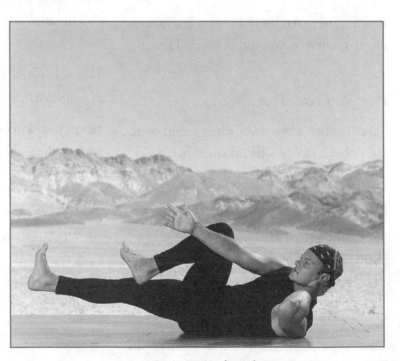

Abdominal Twists (step 2)

5. Extend your left leg and twist to the right side, holding for five breaths.
6. Come back to center and go side to side, eventually taking out the middle pause, and pulse, for a count of thirty.

Connecting Vinyasa

After thirty rotations, come to center and extend the legs up high. With your head and shoulders off the floor, go through your final 60/30 Lift and then release down into the floor.

Pose 24: Supta Baddha Konasana
(page 142)

Bring the soles of your feet together and rest here for ten breaths.

Connecting Vinyasa

When you are ready, bring your knees into your chest and rock-and-roll five times up and back, ending in a seated position with your knees bent and the soles of your feet flat on the floor.

Pose 25: Boat Pose (Navasana)

From the seated position, take Boat Pose three times, following it with the cross-and-lift action each time (see p. 80). Finish in the seated position with the soles of your feet on the floor.

Pose 26: Seated Half Pigeon (Urdhva Mukha Sukhasana)

From the seated position after Boat Pose, cross your right shin over the front of your left thigh and take Seated Half Pigeon (see p. 82). Hold for five breaths.

Pose 27: Three-Legged Tabletop (Arka Purvottanasana)

From Seated Half Pigeon, walk your hands back eight inches with the fingers facing forward and lift your hips up into Three-Legged Tabletop (see p. 82). Drop your head back and hold for five breaths.

Connecting Vinyasa

After five breaths, bring your chin back into your chest and lower your hips down.

Pose 28: Bent Leg Seated Twist (Marichyasana)

Place your right foot down on the floor to the outside of your left knee and take your Bent Leg Seated Twist (see p. 143). Hold for five breaths.

Pose 29: Double Pigeon (Dwapada Rajakapotasana)

Double Pigeon is a powerful stretch that really unlocks and releases the muscles and tissue deep in your hips.

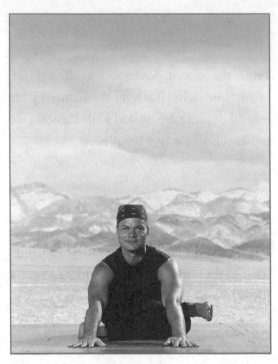

Pose 29: Double Pigeon (Dwapada Rajakapotasana)

4. Walk your hands forward and relax down, letting your head hang forward.
5. Drop your mask and soften your eyes as you breathe deeply.

Alignment

- Stack your shins on top of each other with your legs at right angles.
- Bring the anklebone of the top foot to the outside of the lower thigh.
- Flex your feet.
- Lengthen your spine.

Modification

If you cannot place your upper foot past your lower knee, you can bring your foot to rest inside the knee or take Seated Half Pigeon Pose.

Connecting Vinyasa

After five breaths, come up to sitting and release your legs. Repeat the sequence of Seated Half Pigeon, Three-Legged Table-top, Bent Leg Seated Twist, and Double Pigeon on the left side. After the second Double Pigeon, release your legs and extend them straight out in front of you.

Building Blocks

1. From Seated Twist, bring your lower foot out so the shin is parallel to the front of the mat.
2. Release your right knee down and stack your right shin directly over your left.
3. Place your hands to either side of your hips, pick your body up, and scoot your tail back.

Our hips are the storage depot for our emotions, so deep poses such as these can sometimes feel very intense as you access and release the tension buried there. Breathe way down deep into your pelvis and let the cleansing wind carry away any remaining resistance or tightness you find.

Pose 30: Seated Forward Bend (Paschimottanasana)

Sitting upright, reach underneath your butt and pull your sitting muscles out laterally so you come right onto your sitting bones. Reach forward, hinging at the hips, and take Seated Forward Bend (p. 88).

Connecting Vinyasa

After the tenth breath, inhale and come back up to a seated position.

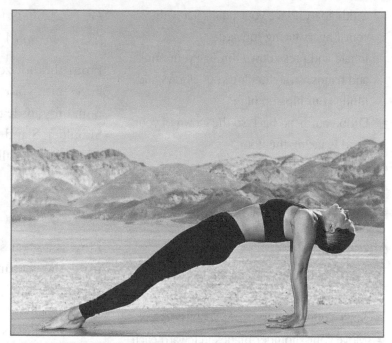

Pose 31: Tabletop (Purvottanasana)

Pose 31: Tabletop (Purvottanasana)

Tabletop neutralizes forward bends and creates an overall feeling of release and expansion.

Building Blocks

1. From a seated position with your legs straight out in front of you, bring your hands back about twelve inches behind your hips, shoulder

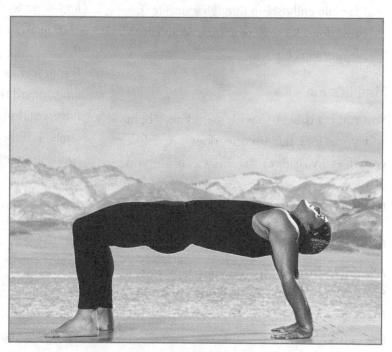

Tabletop (Purvottanasana), modification

width apart. Place your palms flat with your fingers facing forward.

2. Inhale and press down through your arms and hands, straightening your elbows and lifting your hips up high.
3. Drop your head back so the crown of your head is facing the floor.
4. Press all ten toes into the floor.
5. Gaze at the back wall.
6. Breathe deeply and freely for five breaths.

Alignment

- Press your palms and all ten toes down into the floor.
- Stack your shoulders over your wrists.
- Move your shoulder blades in toward each other.
- Maintain enthusiasm through your thighs.
- Press down through your hands and feet to lift your hips higher.

Modification

You can do this pose with your knees bent and your feet flat on the floor (just like your feet in Bridge). In this variation, you want your body from your chest to your knees to be parallel to the floor, like a table.

Connecting Vinyasa

After five breaths, lower your hips to the floor. Extend your legs out straight and lie back onto your mat in preparation for the next pose, Shoulder Stand.

Pose 32: Shoulder Stand (Sarvangasana)

From the horizontal position, bring your knees into your chest and, on the exhalation, lift your legs and hips up to the sky in Shoulder Stand (p. 144). Hold Shoulder Stand for ten full breaths.

Pose 33: Plow (Halasana)

Plow is a great stretch for the entire back, from the sacrum all the way up to the shoulders.

Building Blocks

1. From Shoulder Stand, slowly lower your legs down to the floor behind your head. They may not reach the floor, and that is fine.
2. If your feet touch the floor, bring your arms toward the front wall, interlacing your fingers and squeezing your elbows straight. If they do not, just keep your hands at your lower back for support.
3. Gaze at your navel.
4. Go within and take five soothing, calming breaths.

Alignment

- Keep your head neutral—DO NOT look side to side.
- Walk your shoulder blades in toward each other.
- Press your pubic bone upward.

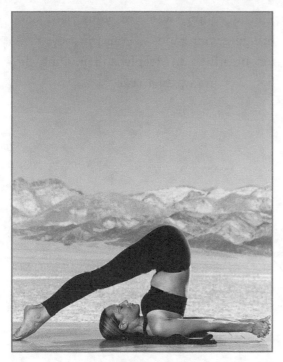

Pose 33: Plow (Halasana)

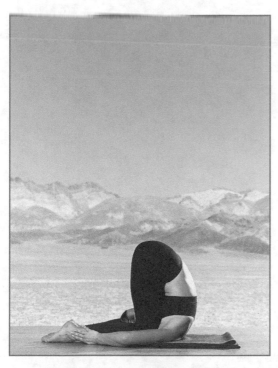

Pose 34: Deaf Man's Pose (Karnapidasana)

- Press your quadriceps toward the ceiling.
- Spin your inner thighs up.

Modification

If it feels too intense to keep your legs straight, bend your knees and place them on your forehead.

Pose 34: Deaf Man's Pose (Karnapidasana)

In this restorative pose, you create sanctuary, deep release, and overall biochemical balance throughout the body.

Building Blocks

1. From Plow, bend and drop your knees in toward your ears.
2. Bring your arms around and take hold of your feet. You can hold the heels, ankles, calves—whatever feels comfortable.
3. You can either point your toes or tuck them under.
4. Stay here for ten to twenty breaths, fully releasing into this profound space-enhancing stretch.

Alignment

- Hold your feet, ankles, or calves.
- Come onto your shoulders.
- Draw your knees in toward your ears.

To finish, do a closing sequence of:

Pose 35: Fish Pose (p. 145)

Pose 36: Supine Twist (p. 116)

Pose 37: Savasana (p. 90)

End by rolling over onto your right side, bringing your hands to your third-eye center, breathing in deeply and inviting the light as you say, "Namaste."

For a quick reference to this week's poses, see page 240.

Week Four Balancing Diet

Abstinence is as easy to me as temperance would be difficult.

—SAMUEL JOHNSON

THROUGHOUT HISTORY, PEOPLE HAVE FASTED FOR DIFFERENT REASONS. SOME FASTED FOR RELIGIOUS REASONS, OTHERS, SUCH AS GANDHI, OUT OF POLITICAL

protest, and some because they knew it was intrinsically good for them. In Week Four, we will do a three-day intensive fruit fast, because active cleansing or fasting is a way to allow your body to fully empty out and get clean, giving your metabolic organs a chance to rest and renew themselves. A lot of people spring-clean their homes, but the same should be done for our bodies now and then as well.

For many years, I did complete fasts, with no food at all. As I've gotten older and have more responsibilities, though, that kind of intense fasting doesn't really feel right anymore. I developed the fruit fast as

a modified way to clean out my system, and then I tried it with my students at bootcamp. For three days in the middle of our weeklong program, we eat nothing but fresh fruit, and the results are amazing. As their bodies shed the toxins that years of poor eating and other bad habits created, they literally start to glow. By removing all that didn't belong, they are able to receive the radiance.

There are always a few people who are worried that they will feel deprived or hungry. Because of our culture of excess, we believe we have to have three big, protein-laden meals a day, otherwise we will

171

be undernourished. But the truth is that we need far less food than we think. By the end of the three days, the students who were the most worried are usually the ones who have the most profound breakthroughs.

I remember one stubborn student who brought a whole bag of protein bars and snacks to Mexico with her because she had no intention of, as she put it, "starving herself for three days." So while the rest of us got lighter, clearer, and brighter over those three days, she kept eating her heavy protein bars and nuts. It was amazing to watch. The whites of everyone's eyes got brighter—all except for hers. The energy in the yoga room grew more buoyant and joyful as they shed layers—except for her. She really stood out in contrast. By the second day, I could tell she regretted her choice, but she was too stubborn to change her mind. At the end of the week, she came up to me and sheepishly admitted that she wished she'd trusted me and the process and done the fruit fast.

"Everyone had these great breakthroughs," she said, "and all I have is a half-finished bag of protein bars and nuts. I can't believe how badly I sabotaged myself here."

"Perhaps," I said, "but maybe this experience did have some value for you. It allowed you to see how you let your brain get in the way of your growth."

"You're absolutely right," she agreed. "And now I'm going to go home and do the fruit fast on my own, so I can feel as good as all these people do!"

If the idea of a three-day cleanse intimidates you, just make up your mind to do it, and you'll see it really isn't a big deal. Also, it helps to remember that avocados and tomatoes are fruits, and there are plenty of things you can do with them in order to feel satisfied.

If you have any health concerns whatsoever that might be triggered by a fruit fast, such as low blood pressure, *please consult your doctor before doing this*. If you are deficient, thin, or weak, you need to be careful to nourish yourself while cleaning out. You will want to supplement your cleanse either with superfoods, such as spirulina, or even one simple small meal a day while cleansing. The process will still be as powerful and totally worthwhile.

Week Four Diet To-Do

The following are the general guidelines for the three-day cleanse:

1. I recommended doing the three-day cleanse at the beginning of the week. From the morning of the first day, eat meals that contain only fruit. It is best to use fresh fruit, but you can also have fruit juices and fruit soups, such as tomato soup, as long as they are natural and additive-free.

2. As often as you can, take the time to prepare full meals, rather than just

grabbing pieces of fruit on the run. Slice up melon and pineapple and arrange them on a plate with some strawberries, blueberries, and blackberries, or any other fruits you like. Make a smoothie with ripe bananas, peaches, and apple juice, and sit down to drink it. Have fun with it; put time and effort into planning your meals, so you feel fulfilled and nourished rather than deprived.

3. Consciously try to fill your time with activities or projects that are not centered around eating. Take a sauna, get a massage, go to the movies, read, go for a walk—whatever nourishes you. For these six days, I suggest eating at home or with people who know and support what you are doing.

4. Meditate!

5. Continue doing your daily yoga practice. At first you may think it is impossible to do sixty minutes of yoga having eaten only fruit, but just try it—I think you will be astonished at what you can do and how you will feel. If you feel weak, simply lower the intensity; stay intuitive.

6. Make sure to really chew your fruit well. This way, you can appreciate the taste more and digest it better; it also promotes better assimilation and elimination.

7. Eat small amounts throughout the day to keep your blood sugar level. If you start to experience any hypoglycemic symptoms, such as headache or dizziness, drink diluted fruit juice to bob your blood sugar back to normal. It takes a lot less than you

A Word About Colonics

If you notice you feel lethargic, foggy in the head, or excessively constipated while you are cleansing, it is because you are releasing toxins and they are floating around in your system. While it is a personal preference, you may want to think about getting a colonic.

If you do decide to get a colonic, be sure to go only to a reputable place, and be sure to limit yourself to two sessions in a period of a year. You can do your two sessions within a week of each other, but more than two colonics in a year upsets the natural order of your system.

Coming Off Your Cleanse

I always tell my students that any fool can fast, but only a wise person can come off it intelligently. It is *very important* that you do not rush out and gorge yourself; otherwise you will experience stomach distress. Just add back in the fresh foods you have been eating all along, *in moderation*. The focus of the next week is centering, and we will talk more there about grounding and bringing your body back into full balance after a radical cleanse, but for the remaining four days of this week, eat simply, plainly, and with full consciousness.

think to keep you steady (remember the wounded Egyptian soldier who was back on his feet with just a little bit of sugar).

8. Drink water, diluted fruit juice, or herbal tea throughout to stay completely hydrated. Stay away from caffeinated beverages. If you are constipated, drink a mild herbal laxative tea such as senna, or find one that you like in a health food store.

Week Four Restoration Meditation
20 Minutes

IT IS DIFFICULT, IF NOT IMPOSSIBLE, TO RE-STORE OURSELVES WHILE WE ARE CAUGHT UP IN THE BUSYNESS OF OUR MINDS. THIS WEEK, WE WILL DO A VERY SIMPLE MEDI-tation to notice how often we get lured into the activity in our minds, away from the stillness that makes true rest and regeneration possible.

Get comfortable and anchor your mind to the now moment. Resolve to let your mind appear as a blank screen for twenty minutes. Watch carefully for thoughts to arise. They may come up as images, tunes, ideas, or words. Some may arise as or with feelings, emotions, or sounds, perhaps in the form of voices. Note the ceaseless images in your mind and how relentlessly they appear to distract you from being still and restoring in quiet.

Do not struggle to free yourself from musical impressions or entertaining or distracting mental noise and chatter. As soon as you become aware of having fallen into the dream stuff—of having been lured away into busyness—step back into the gap between you and your thoughts and let the thoughts go. You may need to do this again and again and again, but that is just what meditation is: beginning again.

The point of meditation is to train ourselves to know the difference between thinking and being lost in thought. If we don't know the difference, we get lost in worlds that exist only inside our heads, and we miss out on the truth and curative beauty of seeing life through a clear lens of present-moment consciousness.

Sit in this restorative meditation for twenty minutes each morning and twenty minutes each evening.

Restoration Excavation Questions

1. What excess baggage am I carrying around with me? What thoughts, feelings, worries, or past situations am I clinging to that drain me?

2. What do I most need to let go of? What are the things that I would be relieved to finally release? Anger toward someone in my life? Stress about money? Fears that arose from a past negative experience?

3. Do I really give myself enough time to relax and restore myself? How can I carve out more time for this?

Week Five: Centering

THERE IS A STORY OF A DISCIPLE WHO ONE DAY CAME TO VISIT HIS MASTER TO ASK IF HE COULD RECEIVE HIS HIGHER RANKING AS A MONK. AS THE DISCIPLE ENTERED THE

temple, he left his shoes and rice bowl outside. The master asked his student, "On which side of the rice bowl did you place your shoes?"

"What kind of nonsense question is that?" asked the student. He was very annoyed. "Why don't you ask me about all the enlightenment I am receiving in meditation, my kundalini rising, and my knowledge of God? I am an advanced student of scripture and meditation—why do you ask me such a stupid and ordinary question?"

Once again the master asked the same question. "On which side of the rice bowl did you place your shoes?"

The angry student replied, "What do rice bowls and shoes have to do with spirituality? Frankly, I take pride in not being overly careful about small things like that. I simply don't remember, because it isn't important."

"You are not ready to graduate to the next level," said the master. "Go and meditate for another nine years, then you can come back and try again."

"Nine years?" said the student. "Just for this small mistake?"

"This is not a small mistake," replied the master. "You are not yet living from your center, because you have no awareness of what is right in front of you. You are not present in your everyday activities, and that is what it means to live meditatively—you must learn to have your feet on the ground."

This story illustrates the need to come down out of our heads and become more intuitively competent and mindful of what is happening right in front of us. It does little good to complain about teachers, husbands or wives, parents, bosses, or lovers. We only accentuate our role as victims when we say, "I'd be happier if only he or she were different," or "If only they would get off my back, I wouldn't get so reactive." Most of us have a side that is loyal to the victim within. But these thought systems of blame and self-pity stunt our growth and strain our relationships.

Our emancipation can only come from within, when we decide we no longer want to live this way. By saying, "I will become centered," we become responsible people; we own our lives from the inside. We don't have to wait for others to set us free. As we practice staying centered we discover that we have the capacity to be aware of the little gremlin voices in our heads and that we don't have to get caught up in the illusions of our own story.

For many of us our lives are so filled with intensity that we often miss out on the quiet that affords us a kind of full presence. Much of our lives may have been lived on a roller coaster of drama and crisis. It may have felt awful, but it was certainly never dull. As we get healthier, life can begin to feel a bit normal without all the drama to liven things up. But simply continuing with the flow of this program and keeping faith in a higher power, we soon see that the simple days, in fact, add up to a very rich life.

This week is about learning to stay intuitively grounded, from where you place your rice bowl in relation to your shoes to how you interact with those around you. It is learning to relax and be present with everything in your life, both big and small. Throughout this week, when you do your practices, focus on really being where you are. When you eat, really eat. Really chew, really taste, really smell, really feel the food dissolve into and nourish your being. When you act, act consciously and with directed intention. Make everything you do a practice of meditative awareness. If you can do this, you will see that your meditation practice is not separate from your life. It will no longer be something you do for a period of time in the morning and evening; it will be a way of life. We think that life is a distraction from meditation, but really, life is an occasion for meditation.

Week Five Yoga Practice
75 Minutes

YOU ARE ALREADY FAMILIAR WITH A LOT OF THE SEQUENCES IN THIS WEEK'S PRACTICE, SO IDEALLY, YOU CAN NOW BEGIN TO FLOW WITH MORE GRACE. COMING OFF YOUR

cleanse of last week, you will experience a new lightness in your practice, which will allow you to go deeper into your poses. During my bootcamps, the days following the cleanse are typically filled with personal breakthroughs, both on and off the mat.

Beginning Vinyasa

Open with the three integration poses: Child's Pose (1), Downward Facing Dog (2), and Ragdoll (3). Then do three rounds of Sun Salutation A and three rounds of Sun Salutation B. After the third round of

Sun Salutation B, go through Sun Salutation B again until you are in Warrior I.

Pose 4: Warrior II (Virabhadrasana II)

From Warrior I, open your arms to Warrior II (see p. 79 for Building Blocks and Alignment), squaring your hips and your chest to the side wall. Hold for five to ten breaths.

Connecting Vinyasa

Helicopter your back arm down to the mat and step back into High Push-Up. Go through the steps of vinyasa A until you are in Downward Facing Dog. Lift your right leg to the sky, rolling your hip open, and reach your right foot toward your left shoulder. This puts you in position for the next pose, Flipped Downward Dog.

Pose 5: Flipped Downward Dog

This is not a traditional yoga pose; you won't find it in any of the ancient yogic texts. It is one that arose very spontaneously and naturally as I developed my own style of Baptiste Power Vinyasa Yoga, and I find it adds a nice sense of freedom and lightness. Don't take this pose too seriously; it's meant to be fun!

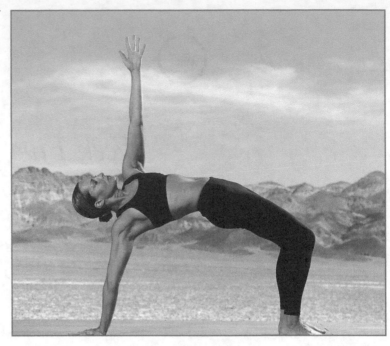

Pose 5: Flipped Downward Dog

Building Blocks

1. With one leg lifted, continue rolling open . . . open . . . open . . . until you just go ahead and flip your dog over, coming onto the soles of your feet and your left palm.

2. Press down in your feet as you lift your hips up high.
3. Extend your right arm up to the sky.
4. Drop your head back and gaze to the front of the room.

Alignment

- Bring your feet a little wider than hip width and parallel.
- Press into the lower hand.
- Lift your hips up high to the sky.
- Let your head drop back.

If you gave this pose to a six-year-old, he or she would have a great time with it. But as grown-ups, we get all caught up in how we look or if we are doing it right. Remember to take your practice seriously, but take yourself lightly.

- To deepen the pose, reach your arm to the front of the room.

Connecting Vinyasa

After five breaths, carefully and mindfully flip back over and come into High Push-Up. In High Push-Up bring your feet and legs together to get ready for the next pose, Side Plank.

Pose 6: Side Plank (Vasisthasana)

Spin your heels to the right and take Side Plank (see p. 105 for Building Blocks and Alignment), left hand up to the sky. Hold for five breaths.

Connecting Vinyasa

Come back to High Push-Up and go through vinyasa A again, ending in Downward Facing Dog. From Downward Facing Dog, bring your right leg up to the sky, bend the upper knee, and externally open the whole front right side of your body. Hold here for a few breaths.

Pose 7: Crescent Lunge (Anjaneyasana)

Square your hips and lunge your raised leg forward to your hands, sweeping up on the inhale into Crescent Lunge (see p. 107 for Building Blocks and Alignment). On the exhale, bring your hands to namaste at your heart center. Take a deep breath in.

Pose 8: Revolving Crescent Lunge (Parivrtta Alanasana)

Exhale and spin your left arm to the outside of your right thigh, coming into Revolving Crescent Lunge (see p. 126 for Building Blocks and Alignment). Hold for five breaths.

Pose 9: Extended Side Angle (Utthita Parsvakonasana)

From Revolving Crescent Lunge, exhale and bring your right forearm to the top of your right thigh. Spin your back foot flat and take Extended Side Angle (see p. 128), either with your left arm stretched to the front wall or with your arms bound. Hold here for five breaths.

Connecting Vinyasa

After five breaths, release your upper hand down to the mat and step your front foot back, coming into High Push-Up. Go through the steps of vinyasa A until you are in Downward Facing Dog. Repeat the entire sequence on the left side: Starting with Warrior I, take Warrior II into Flipped Downward Dog, step into High Push-Up, and then roll your heels to the left for Side Plank. Come back to High Push-Up and go through your vinyasa, ending in Downward Facing Dog. Take the left leg up to the sky and step into Crescent Lunge, Revolving Crescent Lunge, and Extended

Side Angle. After the second Extended Side Angle, go through vinyasa A, ending in Downward Facing Dog.

Pose 10: Thunderbolt (Utkatasana)

From Downward Facing Dog, jump or walk forward. Inhale and lift halfway up, then exhale and fold forward into Standing Forward Bend. Bend your knees, dip your hips low, inhale, and sweep your arms up alongside your ears, coming into Thunderbolt (see p. 76 for Building Blocks and Alignment). Hold here for five breaths.

Pose 11: Prayer Twist
(Parivrtta Utkatasana)

From Thunderbolt, bring your hands down into a prayerlike position at your heart, exhale, and spin to the right, coming into Prayer Twist (see page 108 for Building Blocks and Alignment).

Connecting Vinyasa

Hold for five breaths, then hang forward in Ragdoll. Toe/heel your feet to hip width in preparation for Gorilla Pose.

Pose 12: Gorilla Pose (Padhastasana)

Hook the first two fingers of each hand around the big toes, palms facing each other. Inhale and lift halfway up, then ex-hale and fold forward, coming into Gorilla Pose (see p. 130 for Building Blocks and Alignment). Hold for five breaths.

Connecting Vinyasa

After the fifth breath, release your hands and toe/heel your feet back together. Repeat Prayer Twist to the left side, then fold forward again into Gorilla, this time taking the variation of placing your hands all the way under your feet, palms up. After the fifth breath, release your hands, toe/heel your feet back together, and slowly come rolling up to standing. End in Samasthiti.

Pose 13: Eagle Pose (Garudasana)

From Samasthiti, sweep your arms up overhead and take Eagle Pose (p. 131), two times on each side. End in Samasthiti.

Pose 14: Standing Leg Raise, Front
(Utthita Hasta Padangusthasana A)

Like all single-leg standing poses, this tones and hones the entire standing leg. It is a balancing pose that requires a fixed gaze and steady, equanimous vision.

Building Blocks

1. From Samasthiti, bring your hands together at namaste and gaze down at your fingertips. Take a moment to breathe here and center yourself.

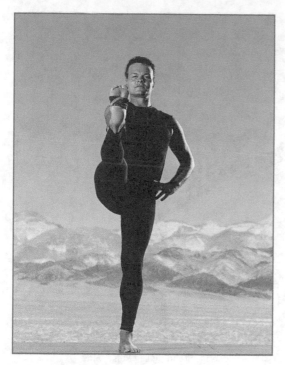

Pose 14: Standing Leg Raise, Front
(Utthita Hasta Padangusthasana A)

5. Inhale and unhinge your knee to whatever degree you can while still maintaining a straight spine.
6. Engage your abdominal lock to stabilize this pose.
7. Keep your eyes fused to a point and stay here for five breaths.

Alignment

- Keep your standing leg strong and straight.
- Keep both buttocks and hips level.
- Maintain a straight spine. (This is more important than a straight leg, so if you are rounding your back, you know you've extended your leg too far.)
- Contract your belly inward.
- Keep your shoulders on one plane; do not turn your torso.

Modification

Work with a bent knee.

Pose 15: Standing Leg Raise, Side (Utthita Hasta Padangusthasana B)

This pose is similar to Standing Leg Raise, Front, and has much of the same strengthening and toning effects. In addition, it

2. When you are ready, bring your gaze forward, locking your eyes on to a fixed spot ahead of you.
3. Bring your right knee up into your chest. Hold the knee with both hands. Place your left hand on your left hip. If you are new at this, stay here. Otherwise, continue.
4. Place your left hand on your left hip and grab your right big toe with the first two fingers of the right hand.

Don't look for perfect poses; that's craziness. It robs you of any joy in the movement. Healthy poses, yes. Perfect poses, not important. The ideal of a pose is something to work toward, not a measuring stick to beat yourself up with.

also opens and strengthens the hip and pelvic muscles.

Building Blocks

1. From Standing Leg Raise, Front, open your right leg (or knee, if you are working with your knee bent) out to the right side.
2. Turn your head and look over your left shoulder.

Alignment

Same as for Standing Leg Raise, plus:

- Drop your right hip down in line with your left.
- Set your eyes over your left shoulder.

Modification

Work with the knee bent. If you need help with balance, extend your left arm towards the left wall like a wing.

Connecting Vinyasa

Bring the extended leg and gaze back to center. Release the toe or knee and place your hands on your hips. Extend the leg out straight, point your toes, and take five full breaths. Then bend your extended leg. This puts you in position for the next pose, Airplane.

Pose 16: Airplane (Dekasana)

Airplane is another one-leg balancing pose, yet it uses every muscle of the body to achieve stability and lightness.

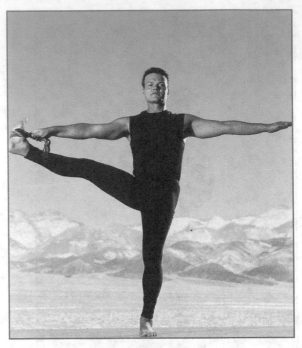

Pose 15: Standing Leg Raise, Side
(Utthita Hasta Padangusthasana B)

Building Blocks

1. From the ending position after Standing Leg Raise, Side, bring both hands to your hips.
2. In one fluid motion, bend the knee, exhale as you hinge forward, and extend your right leg out behind you.
3. Open your arms out behind you like wings with your palms facing down.
4. Arch your back very slightly, bringing a little of the Upward Facing Dog motion into this pose.
5. Lower your chin toward your chest so your neck is neutral and happy.
6. Gaze at the floor about two feet in front of your standing foot.

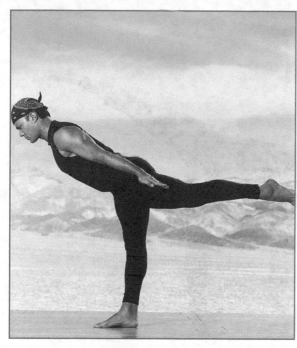

Pose 16: Airplane (Dekasana)

Alignment

- Squeeze your legs and root down through the standing foot.
- Spiral the inner thigh of the raised leg upward and the outer thigh downward.
- Keep your upper foot active.
- Square your hips down to the floor.
- Extend your chest plate forward, creating traction through your torso.
- Keep your chest slightly higher than your hips.

- Draw your shoulder blades down your back.
- Pull your arms back through your fingertips.

Connecting Vinyasa

After five breaths in Airplane, bring your hands to your heart center, pressing your palms together. Keep your upper leg raised. This puts you in position for the next balance pose.

Pose 17: Half Moon (Ardhachandrasana)

This pose is the final one in this balancing sequence of poses. Your muscles will be reaching fatigue, so you need to stay connected with your breath and stay in your center.

Building Blocks

1. With your hands at namaste, reach your left hand down to the floor, about eight inches in front of your left foot. You can press your hand flat or come onto a claw of five fingers.
2. Place your right hand on your hip.
3. Roll your right hip open.

If your practice is about performance, you are guaranteeing weaknesses in your body, because your strong side will only get stronger and your weak side will only get weaker. Your more flexible side will get longer, but your blocked side will get tighter. Why? Because if you are performing, your ego will never let you expose your weaknesses and blocks.

4. Extend the upper leg up to the ceiling.
5. Reach the upper arm straight up.
6. Look up and over your right shoulder.

Alignment

- Press into the standing leg.
- Roll the inner thighs out and away from each other.
- Extend the upper hand directly above the upper shoulder.

Modification

You can use a block under your hand to give yourself more height. If balance is difficult, keep looking down at the floor.

Connecting Vinyasa

After five breaths, release your raised leg down and hang forward in Ragdoll. Rest here for a few breaths, then repeat the sequence of Standing Leg Raise, Front, Standing Leg Raise, Side, Airplane, and Half Moon with your left leg raised. Come back to

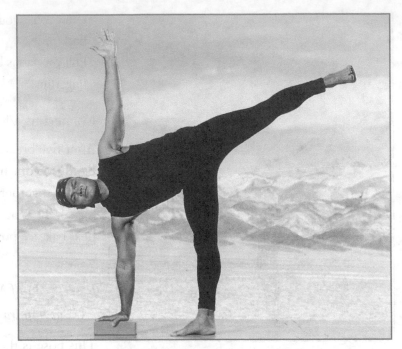

Pose 17: Half Moon (Ardhachandrasana)

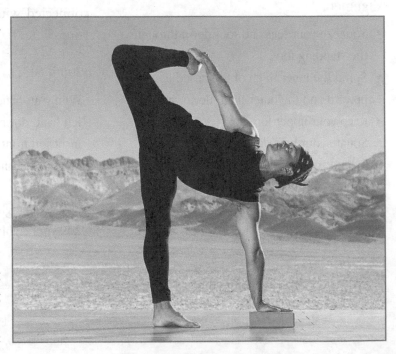

Half Moon (Ardhachandrasana), variation

For a more advanced variation, you can take Bound Half Moon. This pose is very challenging but develops an amazing level of coordination and balance. It requires a good level of skillful focus and whole-body integration.

From Half Moon, bend the knee of the raised leg and grasp the upper foot with the lifted hand. As in bow poses, press actively through the upper leg, bringing the upper knee toward the wall behind you until you get a great stretch through the front side of the upper hip flexor muscles. Open your chest, turn your head, and look upward.

Ragdoll and rest for a few breaths, then come slowly rolling up to standing.

Pose 18: Tree Pose (Vrksasana)

From the standing position, sweep your arms up overhead and take Tree Pose (p. 134).

Connecting Vinyasa

After Tree Pose on each leg, fold forward and go through vinyasa A until you are in Downward Facing Dog.

Pose 19: Triangle (Trikonasana)

Step your right foot forward, coming into Warrior I, then Warrior II. Straighten your right knee on track and reach your right arm forward, taking Triangle Pose (see p. 104).

Connecting Vinyasa

After the fifth exhalation, inhale and let your raised arm pull you up to standing.

Pose 20: Twisting Triangle (Parivrtta Trikonasana)

This deep twisting pose squeezes and rinses all the organs and tissues of your midbody, including your digestive system.

Building Blocks

1. From the standing position after Triangle Pose, step your back foot in a little and turn it in to a 45-degree angle.
2. Bring your hands to your hips and square your hips to the wall in front of you. Really take the time to center your hips, because they will be your anchor in this pose.
3. Bring your left arm up next to your ear.
4. Inhale and reach way up through your left hand.
5. Bend your front knee.
6. Exhale and hinge forward from your hips, placing the left palm on the floor to the outside of your right foot (or to the right shin, foot, or on a block—whatever feels stable).
7. Use your hand to pull your right hip back in line with your left.

8. Straighten the front leg as your pull the right hip back.

9. Inhale and lengthen the spine; exhale and roll the right shoulder back, opening the torso to the side wall.

10. Extend the right arm straight up.

11. Gaze at your upper hand.

Alignment

- Engage powerful legs.
- Square your hips forward.
- Bring your inner thighs together.
- Lift your belly up and in.
- Work a straight line through your spine.
- Shoulders at hip height.
- On the inhale, elongate your spine. On the exhale, twist open.
- Twist from your hips, using them as a steering wheel.
- Press your sitting bones back away from your head.
- Drop your shoulder blades down and spread them apart.
- Line up your arms along a vertical plane and reach through the upper fingertips.
- Relax your face.

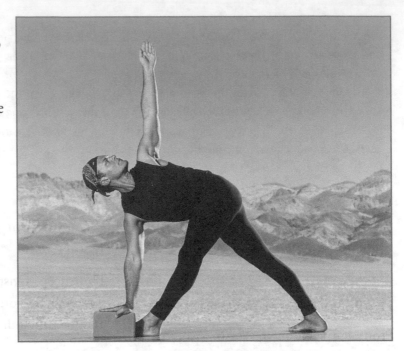

Pose 20: Twisting Triangle (Parivrtta Trikonasana)

Modification

You can use a block to the outside of your front foot, or lift your back heel, to allow you to get more leverage in your twist. You can also lift your back heel off the floor to help you roll your torso open.

Connecting Vinyasa

After five breaths in Twisting Triangle, engage your abdominal lock and helicopter your left arm up and around, pivoting your body so your hips and chest are facing the side wall. Check that your feet are parallel or pigeontoed. You are now in

Never force a twist! Just revolve around as far as feels healthy for you and work the pose there.

position for the next pose, Standing Straddle Bend D.

Pose 21: Standing Straddle Bend D (Prasarita D)

In this variation of Standing Straddle Bend, as you exhale and hinge forward from the hips, slide your hands down your thighs and grab the big toes of each foot with the first two fingers of each hand. Inhale and lift halfway up, then exhale and fold forward, using your finger-to-toe hold as leverage. Hold here for five breaths, working the crown of your head down toward the floor.

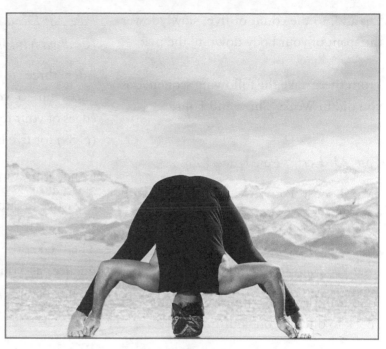

Pose 21: Standing Straddle Bend D (Prasarita D)

Connecting Vinyasa

After five breaths, press into your feet, lengthen your spine, and come back up to standing.

Pose 22: Pyramid Pose (Parsvottanasana)

From Standing Straddle Bend, open your right foot to face the front of the room. Take a moment to square your hips and chest to the front of the room. Inhale and lift your chest and chin, exhale, and hinge forward into Pyramid Pose (p. 161), placing your hands on the floor with the fingers facing the back wall and palms flat.

Connecting Vinyasa

After five breaths, change your hand position so your fingers face forward and step back into High Push-Up. Go through vinyasa A again, ending in Downward Facing Dog. Repeat the sequence of Triangle, Twisting Triangle, Standing Straddle Bend D, and Pyramid Pose with your left leg forward. After the second repetition, go through vinyasa A once again, ending in Downward Facing Dog. From Downward Facing Dog, move forward to High Push-

Up and, to the count of five, slowly lower the front of your body down to the mat.

From there, take the following sequence as you did in Weeks Three and Four:

Pose 23: Locust Pose (page 136)

Take Locust Pose two times. End with your cheek to one side on your mat.

Pose 24: Bow Pose (page 137)

Take Bond Pose two times. End with your cheek to one side on your mat.

Pose 25: Camel Pose (page 109)

Take Camel Pose two times, resting in Downward Facing Dog in between. End in Downward Facing Dog.

Pose 26: Bridge Pose (page 111)

Take Bridge Pose one time, then lower back to your mat. Either repeat Bridge three more times, for a total of four, or take just the one Bridge and then move to Wheel.

Pose 27: Wheel (page 112)

Do Wheel three times, lowering down to your mat in between. Rest with your legs extended out for three to five breaths.

Pose 28: Dead Bug (Urdhva Mukha Upavista Konasana)

After three to five breaths, bring your knees up to your chest, grab the inner edges of your feet, and take Dead Bug Pose (p. 89) for five breaths.

Connecting Vinyasa

After five breaths, release your feet.

Then take the following abdominal sequence, as you did in Weeks Three and Four:

Pose 29: Scissor Legs and 60/30 Lift

Do one set of Scissor Legs, pulsing up for ten breaths, and then one more set, holding up in your highest point for five breaths. Bring both legs to center, extending up to the ceiling, and do one 60/30 Lift. Release your legs to the floor.

Pose 30: Abdominal Twists

Do thirty Abdominal Twists, then bring your legs together and up for one final 60/30 Lift.

Pose 31: Supta Baddha Konasana

Bring the soles of your feet together and rest here for ten breaths. Let your belly drop.

Connecting Vinyasa

When you are ready, bring your knees into your chest and rock-and-roll five times up and back, ending in a seated position with your knees bent and the soles of your feet flat on the floor.

Pose 32: Boat Pose (Navasana)

From the seated position, take Boat Pose five times, taking the cross-and-lift action each time in between (see p. 80). Finish in the seated position with the soles of your feet on the floor.

Pose 33: Upward Facing Boat Pose (Urdhva Padangusthasana)

This variation of Boat Pose releases your skeletal system, allowing for a free whole-body stature as well as building a powerful core and sculpting the muscles of the back, legs, arms, and chest.

Building Blocks

1. From the seated position, grasp the big toes with the first two fingers of each hand.
2. Balancing on your tail and sitting bones, straighten your legs as much as you can.
3. Straighten your spine and both arms.
4. Drop your head back and open your heart to the heavens.
5. Maintain your breath, deep and free.

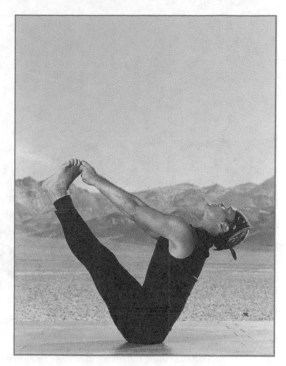

Pose 33: Upward Facing Boat Pose
(Urdhva Padangusthasana)

Alignment

- Keep your legs and feet active.
- Strongly engage your core power to maintain balance.
- Maintain a straight spine.
- Lift and expand your chest.
- Drop your shoulders.
- Relax your face.

Modification

If you would prefer, you can take Easy Boat Pose (p. 114, where you clasp your hands behind bent knees).

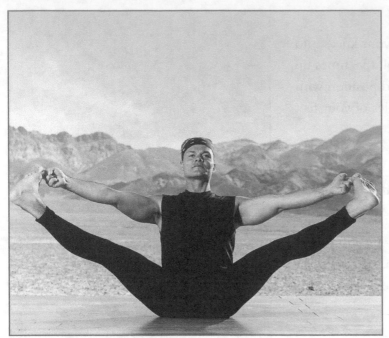

Pose 34: Wide Balancing Boat Pose (Merudandasana)

Pose 35: Seated Half Pigeon (Urdhva Mukha Sukhasana)

From the seated position after Boat Pose, cross your right shin over the front of your left thigh and take Seated Half Pigeon (p. 82). Hold for five breaths.

Pose 36: Three-Legged Tabletop (Arda Purvottanasana)

From Seated Pigeon, walk your hands back eight inches with the fingers facing forward. With your leg still crossed, lift your hips up into Three-Legged Table-top. Hold for five breaths. After five breaths, bring your chin back into your chest and lower your hips down.

Pose 37: Bent Leg Seated Twist (Marichyasana)

Place the sole of your right foot down on the floor, tuck your left foot into your right hip, and twist through your torso with your left elbow pressing into the outside of the right knee.

Pose 34: Wide Balancing Boat Pose (Merudandasana)

This pose opens the hips, strengthens the legs, and develops coordination, balance, and composure.

Building Blocks

While still grasping the big toes with the first two fingers, bring your legs wide apart and away from each other.

Alignment

Same as for Upward Facing Boat Pose.

Pose 38: Double Pigeon (Dwapada Rajakapotasana)

From the neutral position after the Bent Leg Seated Twist, scoot your left foot out so the shin is parallel to the front of the mat. Release your right knee down, stacking your right shin over your left, coming into Double Pigeon (p. 165). Breathe deep for five cleansing breaths.

Connecting Vinyasa

After five breaths, come up to sitting and release your legs. Repeat the sequence of Seated Pigeon, Three-Legged Tabletop, Bent Leg Seated Twist, and Double Pigeon on the left side. After the second Double Pigeon, release your legs and extend them straight out in front of you.

Pose 39: Seated Forward Bend (Paschimottanasana)

Sitting upright, reach underneath your butt and pull your sitting muscles out laterally so you come right onto your sitting bones. Reach forward, hinging at the hips, and take Seated Forward Bend (p. 88).

Connecting Vinyasa

After the tenth breath, inhale and come back up to a seated position.

Pose 40: Tabletop (Purvottanasana)

Walk your hands about eight inches behind you, fingertips facing forward, and on the inhalation, press down through your hands and feet and lift your hips up into Tabletop (see p. 167). Drop your head back and take five breaths here.

Connecting Vinyasa

After five breaths, lower your hips to the floor. Extend your legs out straight and lie back onto your mat in preparation for the next pose, Shoulder Stand.

Next, you can either take Shoulder Stand or Headstand (see Building Blocks and Alignment below).

Pose 41: Shoulder Stand (Sarvangasana)

From the horizontal position, bring your knees into your chest and, on the exhalation, lift your legs and hips up to the sky in Shoulder Stand (p. 144). Hold Shoulder Stand for ten full breaths.

Connecting Vinyasa

After ten breaths, slowly lower down, vertebra by vertebra, until you are lying flat on your mat.

Or

Pose 42: Headstand (Sirsasana)

Headstand is considered one of the most important and powerful yogic postures. It brings a rejuvenating blood flow to the brain, stimulating biochemical and hormonal balance. By turning your world upside down, you give your life new perspective.

Building Blocks

Step One

1. Come into Downward Facing Dog.
2. Bring your knees to the floor, then bring your forearms to the floor. You may want to double up your mat or use a folded blanket to pad your head and arms.
3. Bring each hand to the opposite bicep in order to establish the correct distance between your elbows. Your elbows should be directly under your shoulders. Correct arm placement is key throughout the duration of headstand.
4. Interlace your fingers fully, including the thumbs.
5. Form your hands into the shape they would be in if they were holding a tennis ball. The bottom of both little fingers should be the foundation of the cup that you've formed with your hands.
6. Make sure that the overall shape of your forearms and hands is a symmetrical, equilateral triangle. *Never place your head on the floor without first establishing the correct arm position.*

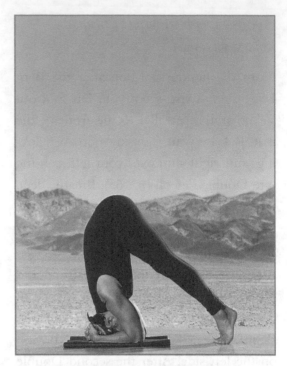

Pose 42: Headstand (Sirsasana), step 1

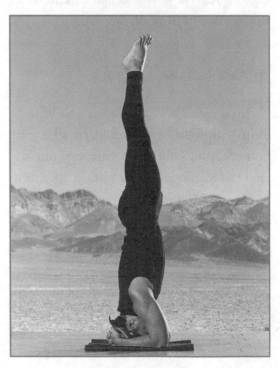

Headstand (Sirsasana), step 2

7. Press your arms downward and lift your shoulders upward and away from each other, broadening your upper back.

Step Two

8. Place the crown of your head on the floor with your skull up against the cup formed by your hands.
9. Gaze straight ahead at your knees and lift your tail.

Step Three

10. Push up on the balls of your feet and straighten your knees.
11. Walk your feet toward your head until your hips are stacked over your shoulders and the back of your body forms a vertical line from your head to your hips. When the weight of your body comes straight down through the center of the crown of your head, the pose will feel effortless and weightless, and there will be no strain on your neck.
12. Pause here and get used to the feel of this position.
13. Exhale and bring your knees into your chest, pushing your legs up off the floor. This action is a bit of a hop, giving you the thrust to raise your legs.
14. Tuck your heels toward your buttocks.

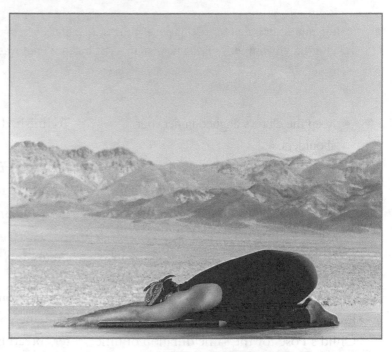

Headstand (Sirsasana), step 3

Step Four

15. Press your arms and shoulders down into the mat.
16. Straighten your knees and bring your whole body into a vertical line.
17. Hold for ten to twenty breaths.

Alignment

- Ground down through the arms and wrists so they take root.
- Remain sensitive to the sensations of weight and pressure on your head and neck.
- Keep your eyes open and gaze straight ahead.
- Keep your shoulder blades broad and away from your ears.

- Keep the elbows aligned under your shoulders.
- Draw your abdominals inward.
- Engage your thighs and rotate them in.
- Press your thighbones backward and your tailbone forward.

Connecting Vinyasa

After ten to twenty breaths in Headstand, lower down into Child's Pose. Stay in Child's Pose for the same duration of time that you were in Headstand.

To finish, do a closing sequence of:

Pose 43: Fish Pose (p. 145)

Pose 44: Supine Twist (p. 116)

Pose 45: Savasana (p. 90)

End by rolling over onto your right side, bringing your hands to your third-eye center, breathing in deeply, and inviting the light as you say, "Namaste."

For a quick reference to this week's poses, see page 243.

Week Five Balancing Diet

If we could give every individual the right amount of nourishment and exercise,
not too little and not too much, we would have found the safest way to health.

—HIPPOCRATES

THERE IS A LOT OF TALK THESE DAYS OF BEING GROUNDED, BUT WHAT DOES THAT REALLY MEAN?

THE ROOT OF THE WORD *GROUND* COMES FROM GERMAN, DUTCH,

and Danish words, all meaning *"bottom,"* particularly of the sea. To be grounded literally means to be in a deep and still place. It means centering down and being fully present, fully stable, fully sane. After the fruit fast, you probably feel very light and clean—maybe even a little raw—and definitely in need of some grounding.

After three days of a fruit fast, you are now fully cleansed and, on the excessive/deficient continuum, in need of some healthy rebuilding. A lot of people, as I said in Week Four, rush right out after a cleanse and gorge themselves on whatever they were missing the most, but that is the nu-

tritional equivalent of walking across a newly cleaned floor with muddy sneakers. All the good you just did is wiped out in an instant if you don't rebuild the right way.

One of the most important things we can do to ground our bodies is to give them minerals. We hear a lot about minerals, but how many of us really know why they are so important? Minerals are of the earth, and to that end, they are quite literally grounding. They make up the whole basis of our core being, because they build our bones. Our bones are the densest and deepest form of our physical selves—they are our structure and our foundation.

Things that rob our bones and bodies of minerals:

Coffee	Too much salt
Refined sugar	Too much protein
Soda and other soft drinks	Anger
Alcohol	Fear
Smoking	Reactivity

Bones are made of minerals, but all the stress and empty foods our culture eats leach these valuable minerals right out of them. In our flighty and excessive world, there is an epidemic of mineral deficiency, which is why diseases such as osteoporosis are so prevalent. We need to reground ourselves by giving our bones the sustenance they need to hold strong and carry us through life.

Week Five Diet To-Do

This week, as you slowly start to add healthful foods back into your diet, concentrate on high-mineral foods. Here are some foods that are especially packed with these vital nutrients:

Whey protein
Seaweed (such as hijiki or nori)
Leafy greens (organic greens have more minerals)
Nuts
Fish (especially halibut, mackerel, sardines)
Root vegetables
Tofu
Broths (chicken or vegetable)
Fresh vegetable or fruit juice

As you eat these life-giving foods, take a few moments to think about your bones. We hardly ever practice gratitude for a part of our body unless it just recovered from an injury, but your bones do so much for you. There is something deeply satisfying about imagining how you are nourishing them in return for all the support and sustenance they have given you throughout your lifetime.

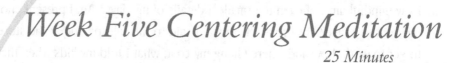

Week Five Centering Meditation

25 Minutes

IN MEDITATION WE EXPERIENCE A CENTER-ING DOWN, A CALMING OF THE USUAL FLOOD AND FLURRY OF THOUGHTS. AS WE SIT THIS WEEK, OUR INTENTION IS TO connect to the symbolic anchors of our hands, body, and breath, thus experiencing the truth that our center is always there, steady and waiting, no matter what swirls up around us.

Begin your practice this week by closing your eyes and bringing your attention to your hands. Observe them gently, anchoring your attention to them and noticing how they begin to tingle with warmth. As distracting thoughts arise, let them go. Do not strain; remember, right aim and right energy. Don't judge yourself if thoughts arise. Don't analyze what or why you are thinking, or build a story around the thoughts. Don't follow your thoughts into the stream-of-dream stuff. If you do, simply pull back into the gap between you and your thoughts and reanchor to your hands, your body, your breath, and the present moment. Each time you get lost in your thoughts, practice the powerful act of coming back to the center and beginning again.

This week, sit in this anchoring meditation for twenty-five minutes each morning and twenty-five minutes each evening.

1. How much do I believe in myself, and how much does this play out in my everyday life? Do I trust my intuition? If so or if not, what results does that produce?

2. When, where, and with whom do I feel the most grounded? With my friends? When I am by myself? With my spouse?

3. How mindful am I of even the smallest details of my days? Am I present enough to notice all the actions I take? Do I remember what I said to the salesperson at the store, what route I took to get to work, how and where I hung my coat, what I told my kids when they asked me a question? Am I truly there in all these moments?

Week Six: Triumph

IN THE FINAL DAYS OF EVERY BOOTCAMP,
AND EVEN IN THE LAST FEW HOURS OF WEEKEND WORK-
SHOPS, THERE IS A SENSE OF VICTORY IN THE AIR. THE STUDENTS WHO

showed up just days before feeling tired, burdened, and tightly wound are now brighter, lighter, and more alive. I look around the room and never fail to be amazed at the power of the process.

Ideally, one part of triumph is coming back to your naturalness. The ancient philosopher Heraclitus once said, "Man is most himself when he achieves the seriousness of a child at play." Our personal victory here in these final five days is about becoming more child*like* and letting go of any child*ish* ways that stop us from entering the kingdom of heaven in our own hearts.

Our willingness to be reinvented is precisely how we let go of our childish ways. In my own process, I had to learn this lesson in order to grow. In popular culture, being a man usually means being a tough guy who shows no emotion and who has sexual power. The media reinforces these deadening attitudes relentlessly, and for many years I posed as who I was "supposed" to be. At a certain point, I recognized that I was buying into a lie and that this was not how I wished to live. I realized it was braver to expose my insecurities rather than to hide them, that it took more strength to connect to people than to control them, more "manhood" to live by thought-out principles rather than in a trancelike compulsion. I found that the real toughness was living from my soul and not my muscles or an immature "macho" mind. I had to give up my childish notions of power and become childlike in order to grow up. I realized that truly courageous men know themselves.

This was a new mind-set for me, and it began a snowballing of breakthroughs, some great, many small. But each breakthrough was a victory for me. The real triumph for us as sannyasins is the many mini-transformations along the way. Jesus said, "Be therefore transformed by the renewing of your mind from within." Truly, the great spiritual triumph is our willingness to mentally renew, change, and grow continually throughout the many seasons of our lives.

Your completion of the forty days is not the end of anything. It is only the beginning of a flexible life, where you can find triumph in staying open to growing and transforming. Somewhere along the way, we get to the point where we need to share our experience. Like I always tell my students as they pack up to go home from a bootcamp, it is not enough just to shine—

we have to go out in the world and share the shine if it is to mean anything. Eventually, we come to see how rich life can be when we share what has worked for us.

Sharing the shine spreads the abundance and also ultimately reflects the light back to us. There is a story of a corn farmer who took first prize every year at the state fair. Each year he shared his prize-winning seeds with all the other farmers in his community. Somebody asked him, "Why do you share your best corn with everyone? You are creating your own competition!"

"Really, it's a matter of self-interest," he replied. "You see, the wind picks up the pollen and carries it from field to field, so if my neighbors grow inferior corn, the cross-pollination lowers the quality of my own corn. That is why I am concerned that they plant only the very best."

As you go through your practices for these remaining five days, remember that triumph happens in the small things. The many small victories of growth accumulate into great ones. Triumph is sharing rather than clinging to success, dissolving the rocks in our minds one by one, discovering the potent value of stillness, and seeking the truth in all things. This is the lifelong path to lightheartedness.

Week Six Yoga Practice
90 Minutes

YOU'VE MADE IT TO THE FINAL PRACTICE!
IN THESE LAST FIVE DAYS OF YOUR PROGRAM, YOU WILL
DO A FULL NINETY-MINUTE YOGA PRACTICE, SIMILAR TO WHAT I TEACH

at my studios.

Beginning Vinyasa

Open with the three integration poses: Child's Pose (1), Downward Facing Dog (2), and Ragdoll (3). Then do four rounds of Sun Salutation A and three rounds of Sun Salutation B. After the third round of Sun Salutation B, go through the steps of Sun Salutation B again until you are in Warrior I.

Pose 4: Warrior II (Virabhadrasana II)

From Warrior I, open your arms up to Warrior II (see p. 79 for Building Blocks and Alignment). Hold for five breaths.

Connecting Vinyasa

Helicopter your arms down to the mat and step back into High Push-Up. Go through the steps of vinyasa A until you are in Downward Facing Dog. Lift your right leg to the sky, rolling your hip and torso open.

Pose 5: Flipped Downward Dog

With your right leg lifted, continue rolling open until you flip over into Flipped Downward Dog. Breathe here for the count of five.

Connecting Vinyasa

After five breaths, carefully and mindfully flip back over and come into High Push-Up. In High Push-Up bring your feet and legs together to get ready for the next pose, Side Plank.

Pose 6: Side Plank (Vasisthasana)

From Downward Facing Dog, move forward into High Push-Up, spin your heels to the right, and take Side Plank (see p. 105 for Building Blocks and Alignment). Hold for five breaths.

Connecting Vinyasa

Come back to High Push-Up and go through vinyasa A again, ending in Downward Facing Dog. From Downward Facing Dog, bring your right leg up to the sky, bend the upper knee, and externally open the whole front right side of your body. Hold here for a few breaths.

Pose 7: Crescent Lunge (Anjaneyasana)

Square your hips and lunge your raised leg forward to your hands, sweeping up on the inhale into Crescent Lunge (see p. 107 for Building Blocks and Alignment). On the exhale, bring your hands to namaste at your heart center. Take a deep breath in.

Pose 8: Revolving Crescent Lunge (Parivrtta Alanasana)

Exhale and spin your left arm to the outside of your right thigh, coming into Revolving Crescent Lunge (see p. 126 for Building Blocks and Alignment). Hold for five breaths.

Pose 9: Extended Side Angle (Utthita Parsvakonasana)

From Revolving Crescent Lunge, exhale and helicopter up to Warrior II. Place your right forearm at the top of your right thigh. Spin your back foot flat and take Extended Side Angle (see p. 128), either with your left arm stretched to the front wall or with your arms bound. Hold here for five breaths.

Connecting Vinyasa

After five breaths, release your upper hand down to the mat and step your front foot back, coming into High Push-Up. Go through the steps of vinyasa A until you are in Downward Facing Dog, then repeat the entire sequence on the left side. Starting with Warrior I, take Warrior II into Flipped Dog, step into High Push-Up, and then roll your heels to the left for Side Plank. Come back to High Push-Up and go through your vinyasa, ending in Downward Facing Dog. Take the left leg up to the sky and step into Crescent Lunge, Revolving Crescent Lunge, and Extended Side Angle. After the second Extended Side Angle, go through vinyasa A, ending in Downward Facing Dog (2).

Pose 10: Thunderbolt (Utkatasana)

From Downward Facing Dog, jump or walk forward. Lift halfway up, then fold forward into Standing Forward Bend. Bend your knees, drop your hips, inhale, and sweep your arms up alongside your ears, coming into Thunderbolt (see p. 76 for Building Blocks and Alignment). Hold here for five breaths.

Pose 11: Prayer Twist
(Parivrtta Utkatasana)

From Thunderbolt, bring your hands down into a prayerlike position at your heart, exhale, and spin to the right, coming into Prayer Twist (see page 108 for Building Blocks and Alignment).

Connecting Vinyasa

Hold for five breaths, then fold forward into Ragdoll (3). Toe/heel your feet to hip width in preparation for Gorilla Pose.

Pose 12: Gorilla Pose (Padhastasana)

Hook the first two fingers of each hand around the big toes. Inhale and lift halfway up, then exhale and fold forward, coming into Gorilla Pose (see p. 130 for Building Blocks and Alignment). Hold for five breaths.

Connecting Vinyasa

After the fifth breath, release your hands and toe/heel your feet back together. Repeat Prayer Twist to the left side, then fold forward again into Gorilla, this time taking the variation of placing your hands all the way under your feet, palms up. After the fifth breath, release your hands, toe/heel your feet back together, and slowly come rolling up to standing. End in Samasthiti (4).

Pose 13: Eagle Pose (Garudasana)

From Samasthiti, sweep your arms up overhead, coming into Mountain Pose (5). From there, take Eagle Pose (p. 131), two times on each side. End in Samasthiti (4).

Pose 14: Standing Leg Raise, Front
(Utthita Hasta Padangusthasana A)

From Samasthiti, take your right big toe (or your knee) with the first two fingers of the right hand, inhale, and extend your leg, coming into Standing Leg Raise, Front (p. 182). Fuse your eyes to a point and stay here for five breaths.

Pose 15: Standing Leg Raise, Side (Utthita Hasta Padangusthasana B)

From Standing Leg Raise, Front, open your right leg (or knee, if you are working with your knee bent) out to the right side. Turn your head so your gaze is to the left wall and stay here for five breaths.

Connecting Vinyasa

Bring the extended leg and gaze back to center. Release the toe or knee and place your hands on your hips. Extend the leg out straight and take five full breaths.

Pose 16: Airplane (Dekasana)

From the ending position after Standing Leg Raise, Side, take a deep breath in, and as you exhale hinge forward into Airplane (p. 184) for five breaths.

Connecting Vinyasa

Bring your hands to your heart center and fix your eyes on one point.

Pose 17: Half Moon Pose (Ardhachandrasana)

With your hands at your heart center, breathe in and then slowly bring your left hand down to the floor for Half Moon Pose.

Connecting Vinyasa

After five breaths, release your raised leg down and hang forward in Ragdoll (3). Rest here for a few breaths, then repeat the sequence of Standing Leg Raise, Front, Standing Leg Raise, Side, Airplane, and Half Moon Pose with your left leg raised. Come back to Ragdoll and rest for a few breaths, then step your left leg back to come into your next pose.

Pose 18: Deep Hip Lunge (Ardha Virabhadrasana)

This is an incredible hip opener as well as an intense strength builder.

Building Blocks

1. Drop your back knee to the floor and place the top of your back foot flat on the floor.
2. Lunge your weight forward into your front knee.
3. Place both hands at the base of your back, fingertips pointing up and arms/elbows wrapped in to shoulder width.
4. Once you are steady, inhale and sweep your arms up to the sky for five breaths.

You might be thinking that this seems like an advanced pose, but there is no such thing as an advanced pose. What advances is the state of your mind.

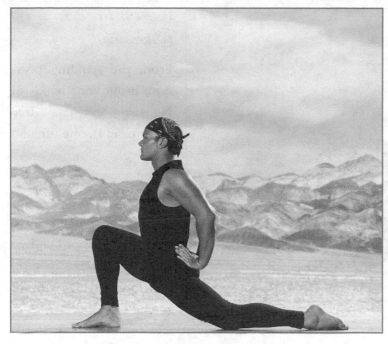

Pose 18: Deep Hip Lunge (Ardha Virabhadrasana), step 1

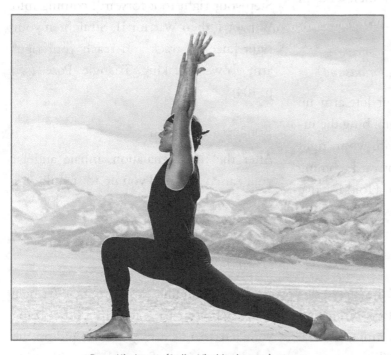

Deep Hip Lunge (Ardha Virabhadrasana), step 2

5. Now comes the intense part: keeping your back foot *exactly* as it is, lift the back knee off the floor. You are pressing the top of your back foot into the floor.

6. Breathe deeply for five breaths.

Alignment

- Point your back foot straight back.
- Let your front knee move forward past your toes (this is the only pose where you do not need to stack your knee over your ankle).
- When you lift your leg, press into the front foot and the top of the back foot.

Connecting Vinyasa

After five breaths, gently lower your back knee to the floor and step back into High Push-Up. Go through vinyasa A up until Downward Facing Dog. Take two deep breaths and then step your right leg back for Deep

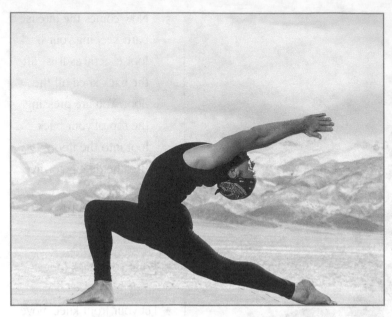

Deep Hip Lunge (Ardha Virabhadrasana), step 3

Pose 20: Tree Pose (Vrksasana)

From the standing position, bring your hands to Namaste and take Tree Pose (p. 134), one time on each leg.

Connecting Vinyasa

After the second Tree Pose, fold forward and go through vinyasa A until you are in Downward Facing Dog.

Hip Lunge. After five breaths, go through vinyasa A once more, and then end in Samasthiti.

Pose 19: Dancer's Pose (Natarajasana)

From Samasthiti, bring your left arm up and bend your right knee, grabbing the inside of your right foot with your right hand. Exhale and launch forward, coming into Dancer's Pose (p. 133). Hold for five breaths, remembering to fuse your gaze to a steady point.

Connecting Vinyasa

After five breaths, release the upper leg down and repeat Dancer's Pose on the left side. Repeat the pose once more on each side, then release into Samasthiti.

Pose 21: Triangle (Trikonasana)

Step your right foot forward, coming into Warrior I, then Warrior II. Straighten your right knee on track and reach your right arm forward, taking Triangle Pose (see p. 104).

Connecting Vinyasa

After the fifth exhalation, inhale and let your raised arm pull you up to standing.

Pose 22: Twisting Triangle (Parivrtta Trikonasana)

From the standing position after Triangle Pose, step your back foot in a little, bring your left arm next to your ear, and on the exhalation hinge forward into Twisting

Triangle (p. 187). Gaze to your upper hand and take five breaths here.

Connecting Vinyasa

After the fifth breath, engage your abdominal lock and helicopter your left arm up and around, pivoting your body so your hips and chest are facing the side wall. You are now in position for the next pose, Standing Straddle Bend D.

Pose 23: Standing Straddle Bend D

Exhale and hinge forward from the hips, sliding your hands down your thighs and grabbing the big toes of each foot with the first two fingers of each hand. Inhale and lift halfway up, then exhale and fold forward, coming into Standing Straddle Bend D (p. 189). Hold here for five breaths, working the crown of your head down toward the floor.

Connecting Vinyasa

After five breaths, press into your feet, lengthen your spine, and come back up to standing.

Pose 24: Pyramid Pose
(Parsvottanasana)

Open your right foot to the front of the room as you square your chest and hips to the front wall. Inhale and lift your chest

and chin; exhale and hinge forward into Pyramid Pose (p. 161).

Connecting Vinyasa

After five breaths, change the position of your hands so your fingers are facing forward and step back into High Push-Up. Go through vinyasa A again, ending in Downward Facing Dog. Repeat the sequence of Triangle, Twisting Triangle, Standing Straddle Bend D, and Pyramid Pose with your left leg forward. After the second repetition, go through vinyasa A once again, ending in Downward Facing Dog. From Downward Facing Dog, move forward to High Push-Up and, to the count of five, slowly lower the front of your body down to the mat.

From there, take the following back-bending sequence, as you did in Weeks Three, Four, and Five:

Pose 25: Locust Pose (page 136)

Take Locust Pose two times. End with your cheek to one side on your mat.

Pose 26: Bow Pose (page 137)

Take Bow Pose two times. End with your cheek to one side on your mat.

Pose 27: Camel Pose (page 109)

Take Camel Pose two times, resting in Downward Facing Dog in between. End in Downward Facing Dog.

Pose 28: Bridge Pose (page 111)

Take Bridge Pose one time, then lower back to your mat. Either repeat Bridge four more times for a total of five, or take just the one Bridge and then move to Wheel.

Pose 29: Wheel (page 112)

Take Wheel four times (once more than last week), lowering down to your mat in between. Rest with your legs extended out for three to five breaths.

Pose 30: Dead Bug
(Urdhva Mukha Upavista Konasana)

After three to five breaths, bring your knees up to your chest, grab the inner edges of your feet, and take Dead Bug Pose (p. 89).

Connecting Vinyasa

After five breaths, release your feet.

Then take the following abdominal sequence, as you did in Weeks Four and Five:

Pose 31: Scissor Legs and 60/30 Lift

Do one set of Scissor Legs, pulsing up for ten breaths, and then one more set, holding up in your highest point for five breaths. Bring both legs to center, extending up to the ceiling, and do one 60/30 Lift. Release your legs to the floor.

Pose 32: Abdominal Twists

Do thirty abdominal twists, then bring your legs together and up for one final 60/30 Lift.

Pose 33: Supta Baddha Konasana

Bring the soles of your feet together and rest here for ten breaths. Let your belly drop.

Connecting Vinyasa

Bring your knees in to your chest and roll them over to one side. Turn your head in the opposite direction and take a deep twisting stretch. Let your arms rest out to the sides. After a few breaths, roll your legs to the other side, then bring your knees into your chest and rock-and-roll five times up and back, ending in a seated position with your knees bent and the soles of your feet flat on the floor.

Pose 34: Boat Pose (Navasana)

From the seated position, take Boat Pose five times, taking the cross-and-lift action each time in between (see p. 80). Finish in the seated position with the soles of your feet on the floor.

Next take the following hip-opening sequence, as you did in Weeks Four and Five:

Pose 35: Seated Half Pigeon (Urdhva Mukha Sukhasana)

From the seated position after Boat Pose, cross your right shin over the front of your left thigh and take Seated Half Pigeon (p. 82). Hold for five breaths.

Pose 36: Three-Legged Tabletop (Arda Purvottanasana)

From Seated Half Pigeon, walk your hands back eight inches with the fingers facing forward. With your leg still crossed, lift your hips up into Three-Legged Tabletop. Hold for five breaths. After five breaths, bring your chin back into your chest and lower your hips down.

Pose 37: Bent Leg Seated Twist (Marichyasana)

Place the sole of your right foot down on the floor, tuck your left foot into your right hip, and twist through your torso with your left elbow pressing away from the right knee.

Pose 38: Double Pigeon (Dwapada Rajakapotasana)

From the neutral position after Bent Leg Seated Twist, scoot your left foot out so the shin is parallel to the front of the mat. Release your right knee down, stacking your right shin over your left, coming into Double Pigeon (p. 165). Breathe deep for five cleansing breaths.

Connecting Vinyasa

After five breaths, come up to sitting and release your legs. Repeat the sequence of Seated Half Pigeon, Three-Legged Tabletop, Bent Leg Seated Twist, and Double Pigeon on the left side. After the second Double Pigeon, release your legs and extend them straight out in front of you.

Pose 39: Seated Forward Bend (Paschimottanasana)

Sitting upright, reach underneath your butt and pull your sitting muscles out laterally so you come right onto your sitting bones. Reach forward, hinging at the hips, and take Seated Forward Bend (p. 88). Hold for ten breaths.

Connecting Vinyasa

After the tenth breath, inhale and come back up to a seated position.

Pose 40: Tabletop (Purvottanasana)

Walk your hands about eight inches behind you, fingertips facing forward, and on the inhalation, press down through your hands and feet and lift your hips up into Tabletop (see p. 167). Drop your head back and take five breaths here.

Connecting Vinyasa

After five breaths, lower your hips to the floor. Extend your legs out straight and lie back onto your mat in preparation for the next pose, Shoulder Stand.

Next, you can take either Headstand or Shoulder Stand, Plow, and Deaf Man's Pose:

Pose 41: Shoulder Stand (Sarvangasana)

From the horizontal position, bring your knees into your chest and, on the exhalation, lift your legs and hips up to the sky in Shoulder Stand (p. 144). Hold here for ten breaths.

Pose 42: Plow (Halasana)

From Shoulder Stand, use your core power to slowly lower the legs down to the floor for Plow (p. 168).

Pose 43: Deaf Man's Pose (Karnapidasana)

After five breaths in Plow, bring your knees in next to your ears for Deaf Man's Pose. Stay here for ten to twenty breaths.

Connecting Vinyasa

When you are ready, slowly lower down, vertebra by vertebra, until you are lying flat on your mat.

Alternate Pose 41: Headstand (Sirsasana)

Come into Downward Facing Dog and go through steps 1 through 3 of the Building Blocks for Headstand (p. 194). Hold here for ten to twenty breaths, then lower down into Child's Pose. Remain in Child's Pose for the same duration of time that you were in headstand.

To finish, do a closing sequence of:

Pose 44: Fish Pose (p. 145)

Pose 45: Supine Twist (p. 116)

Pose 46: Savasana (p. 90)

End by rolling over onto your right side, sitting up, bringing your hands to your third-eye center, breathing in deeply, and inviting the light as you say, "Namaste."

For a quick reference to this week's poses, see page 247.

Week Six Balancing Diet

The chief pleasure in eating does not consist in costly seasoning,
or exquisite flavor, but in yourself.

—HORACE

FROM ANCIENT TIMES RIGHT UP UNTIL TODAY, HARVEST TIME HAS BEEN CAUSE FOR CELEBRATION AND A TIME OF TRIUMPH. HERE, IN THESE FINAL FIVE DAYS OF

your program, you can begin to gather up all the fruits of your efforts and reap the bounty of all you have learned, revealed, and come to appreciate in terms of how you nourish your body.

Week Six Diet To-Do

During these five days, take the time to look back over the past five weeks' worth of eating habits and ask yourself: From which did I most benefit? Which habits and practices yielded the greatest results for me? Which do I want to incorporate into my lifelong eating habits going for-

ward? I encourage you to actually write your responses down somewhere, because as time goes on, it can be easy to forget how good you felt when your diet was in balance and to slip back into old, negative patterns. I see this a lot with students who come to bootcamps. For a few months after returning home, they continue with their healthy habits, but only those who consciously record these results sustain their new habits in the long run. Committing your new plan and way of feeling to paper is a tangible way to keep yourself conscious in this regard.

Having spent the past five weeks bringing your body's ecosystem into balance, you may feel as though you want to incorporate and enjoy some of your old favorite foods. If you love sweets or pizza, you can go ahead and enjoy these things—just remember to use your newly found radar of how much is enough. If your body is clean, balanced, and healthy, it can accommodate foods that might not necessarily be considered nutritious for the body but that feed the soul on another level. Again, it's all about balance. Life is meant to be enjoyed, and food can be a wonderful part of that. Some of my happiest times with my kids are when we stop for ice cream after one of their athletic games, or when we are out for Chinese food. I wouldn't trade those moments or memories for anything.

You can bring the idea of "sharing the shine" into your eating life as well. Breaking bread with others is a very important theme in life. When we sit down together to share nourishing food, nourishing conversation, and nourishing company, we are connecting on a very basic level. We can open new vistas within ourselves and in those around us when the barriers are down and we are communing in this most primal and spiritual of ways. Others may begin to notice the healthy changes within you and may wonder what they can do to get a taste of that. Without proselytizing or saying even a single thing, you may begin to inspire them to make some changes in how they eat. St. John the Divine once said, "Preach all the time; sometimes even with words."

Stay flexible. Continue to try new foods, and stay open and receptive to what your body needs throughout different times of the year. Remind yourself that you are constantly building yourself by what and how much you eat, and at the same time cleansing yourself by the same. Most of all, remember that your physical body is the vehicle that carries you through this life, and the more love and care you put into its maintenance, the sweeter that life will ultimately be.

Week Six Triumph Meditation
30 Minutes

LIKE LIFE, MEDITATION IS A CONSTANT CYCLE OF STILLNESS AND CHAOS, FORGETTING AND RE-MEMBERING. EACH TIME YOU REMEMBER TO COME BACK TO YOUR

breath and let go of the mental distraction is a victory. As time goes by and your practice deepens, you will be able to look back and see that the time between your drifting off and coming back to center gets shorter and shorter. Ultimately, your meditative awareness will become so natural to you that this state of being will become a way of life.

As you become more skillful in not getting involved with your thoughts, you realize that all thoughts have a natural cycle of rising, lingering, and then melting away. You may notice how the thoughts create strong feelings or bodily sensations: ap-

petites, cravings, sexual excitement, physical pain. But as you sit this week, just watch and see how these seemingly powerful sensations rise, swell, and then dissolve and disappear. As the yogic principle of *enicha* says, nothing is permanent—everything will eventually pass. The more we embrace the constant change of life, the less we are knocked over by it. And the less we can be affected by outside forces, the more inner triumph we experience on our spiritual journeys.

In this, your final week, sit for thirty minutes every morning and thirty minutes every evening.

Triumph Excavation Questions

1. On the top of the page, write, "I want to manifest . . ." Then leave four or five lines and write that again. Do this a total of four times. Spend two minutes on each one. Don't censor yourself here—just write down whatever surfaces. Telling your mind allows your intention to take root and blossom.

2. What would you do in your life if you could not fail? Would you change something? Try something new?

3. What are the limiting beliefs that are preventing you from doing what you wrote in question 2? Do you think that you would fail? That you might succeed? That others would be resentful? That you don't have the time, or shouldn't, or aren't "supposed to"?

4. What is your overall life vision?

PART THREE

After the Revolution

The Daily Practices for Living an Awakened Life

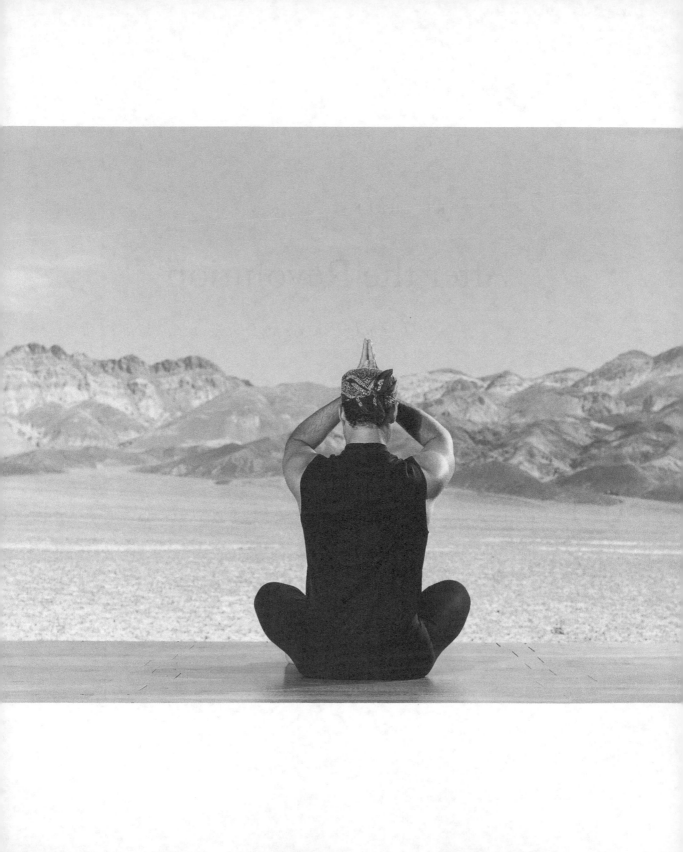

After the Revolution

The Daily Practices for Living an Awakened Life

IN BODY AND SOUL, YOU'VE CHANGED. WHOEVER YOU WERE AT THE BEGINNING OF THESE FORTY DAYS NO LONGER EXISTS; YOU ARE A DIFFERENT PERSON. SO IT

makes sense that you would now want to operate from your new state of mind and health in every moment of your life. This part of the book is meant to take you beyond your revolution, into your personal purpose and way of living.

People often confuse purpose with goals, but they are not the same. I was once having a discussion with a man who was a very well-known self-improvement guru about what it is to live a successful life. He said, "I believe there are certain principles that, if followed, will produce a life of success. The first one is to have clear-cut goals for oneself."

I told him that I had a totally different take on things. For me, living a successful and happy life means not having any goals. "In fact," I said, "the only goal I have is to have no goals."

Of course, he was shocked to hear this, but I went on to explain that at a certain point in my life, I had to ask myself which was more important: my goals or God's goals. My goals were an attempt to manipulate reality in my favor (or so my ego thought). My *purpose,* however, was to be a vessel for good in the world, in whatever form that took. In this way, I could live out God's goals for me.

Really, giving up goals is a high form of faith.

If you look at young children, you'll notice that they have no goals. They tend to be much happier than we are as adults, much more free and light. Why? Because without goals, they can simply relax, be creative, and learn from reality as it is. When we have fixed goals, we are struggling to force things to turn out a certain way. Hence we close ourselves off from seeing what is possible and what else is available to us. We can't see the bigger picture.

So does this mean that we lie down and become doormats? Of course not. It means we walk by faith. We do our work and trust that the visions, the intuitions, and the guidance will come to us. When we ask to be used on behalf of goodness' sake, we may be used for great things. Part of our growth is continuing to get ourselves out of the way so that we can become instruments of a higher power. There is a flow of love, goodness, justice, and compassion in the universe, and we serve that flow not by setting goals based on what we think that flow should be or what it should look like, but by being willing and open vessels through which this flow can manifest itself in the world.

I often get asked by businesspeople what my goals are for my business. "What do you want to create?" they ask. Again, I usually say that I really don't have any goals for my studios and my teaching, except for it to be a ministry that serves humanity. I'm not interested in seeing every person who comes through the door as a potential sale; I am interested in seeing each of them as an opportunity to offer some peace and sanity from the dog-eat-dog mentality that so often confronts us in the world. Rather than get a sale of another product to build our business, I aim to provide a space that people find uplifting. When we give to others with the idea of really serving, without concern for getting, we end up creating something special. You ultimately send out a vibe that will attract people to you and to what you do.

It is hard for businesspeople to understand this, because in today's popular wisdom, we are all programmed to want more. I point out that I am okay with taking one day at a time, one threshold of growth at a time. If a revelation or vision comes to me and rings true as a directive within, I will walk down that path. But I really have no desire to draw out my entire ten-, twenty-, and thirty-year plans of how I want things to turn out, because that kind of vision is limiting. I know that in my life, spiritual growth often takes me in surprising and unexpected directions. My job is to just stay open.

There may be things in my mind that I would like to do, and those things are seedling intentions that will sprout once the proper elements organize themselves in the right ways. If those seeds dry up and blow away, they weren't meant to take root in my life; they were not part of the higher plan for me. This attitude has helped to keep me free and allows me to live in faith. I believe we all need to *discover* our potential, not create it.

It serves no one to strive to *do* better or *do* more. We only grow by seeking to *be* better every day, in every moment, both within ourselves and in the world with those around us. I remember a woman who once told me that she had very tentatively attended her first bootcamp with me over five years earlier. She said she came planning to find out what this whole "personal revolution thing" was all about and use what made sense, but not to get too personally involved with the rest of the participants.

"Thank goodness, growth surprises us with outcomes never expected," she said. This woman learned about the principles that could help her grow in life, but it was the connections she ultimately made with others in the program that showed her how to apply these principles to her daily life. What strikes me as so key about that student's experience is the powerful and necessary combination of humanity and spirituality. We grow and learn not only in isolation, but also through applying our practices to our interactions with people in our daily lives.

I know that in my daily life, I can get caught up in my emotions and in stress. I can lose perspective in the intensity of a stressful situation. Over many years I have developed anchors, or what I call *practices of enlightenment,* that bring me back to my senses. In my life I have repeatedly found that these simple practices can serve as touchstones for sanity and enlightenment in those moments. To have a simple truth that shines light into the difficult moments of my life and that speaks to my heart brings me out of my confusion and serves as an internal reference point that helps me recall what's most important to me.

As you continue on in your journey, I offer you the touchstones of practice that help keep you on a safe and sane path. A touchstone symbolizes the spiritual quality of a solid, unbreakable base. My hope is that the practices of enlightenment serve as touchstones in your life—principles against which to measure yourself, your thoughts, your behavior—and as tangible reminders of truth. I hope they ignite new possibilities in you and strengthen you on your path.

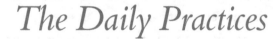

The Daily Practices

The Practice of Preparation

FOR MANY OF US THERE WILL BE TIMES WHEN IT IS HARD TO KEEP TO THE PATH AND STAY TRUE TO AN ONGOING REVOLUTION. THERE WILL BE DIFFICULT MOMENTS,

because that is how life flows. It helps if we can make peace with this truth and accept it, because then we can be more prepared and hold on to our center during tough times.

Having a good set of habits and sticking to them gives us a foundation in our lives. Make it a practice to give time to activities that feed your mind, body, and soul each day. Sticking to your good habits is like keeping a savings account: When challenging times come, you'll have enough accumulated spiritual resources to see you through.

Action to Take

Work a habit that adds to your "body and soul savings account" today. Meditate, practice yoga, get into nature, read something soulful—whatever centers and nourishes you.

The Practice of Compassion

Compassion is a spiritual way of living and walking through life. How we treat all there is in life—ourselves, our bodies, our neighbors, our enemies—matters. Compassion comes through understanding our own sorrow, sadness, emptiness, anger, and fear. Only when we know our own darkness can we be present and compassionate with the darkness that others struggle with.

We can begin the practice of compassion at a very practical level by simply treating ourselves—inside and out, body and soul—and everything around us in a more respectful and honorable way. Many of us have not learned how to do this; we have learned simply to accept pain and abuse, or to be hard-hearted or abusive. With practice, we can learn how to soften our hearts and thus let our selfishness and self-pity drop away.

Action to Take

Start practicing compassion right from where you are. This means holding true to the golden rule of respecting others as you would like to be respected, practicing patience with yourself and others, and reserving harsh words and judgments that serve only to wound. If you do this, very quickly you will notice that your capacity for compassion expands.

The Practice of Being Spontaneous

The practice of letting go of control and excessive planning and instead letting your intuition guide you is a very revolutionary thing to do.

Overcontrol and perfectionism are spiritually deadening. They leave no room for joy or for freedom. When we are in touch with ourselves and with God, we are free to experiment and venture into new territories. We are not in a process of discovery when we simply do the same things correctly again and again. We learn from doing new things in new ways and making mistakes. Spontaneity is trusting our instincts, taking ourselves by surprise, and snatching from the clutches of our well-organized routine a bit of adventure, rather than shying away from it.

Action to Take

Do something spontaneous today. Intuitively speak and act on your feet.

The Practice of Intimacy

Our fear of intimacy is often a fear of getting to know ourselves. We may push intimacy away, or we may completely lose ourselves in another person. Either way, this has kept many of us lonely.

Many of us fear connection and closeness beyond the "fireworks" stage of a relationship. Other times we pursue connection, but when we meet with our own emptiness, we decide that that isn't the right person for us and run in search of a new excitement. If we really haven't gotten to know ourselves, we will always struggle with how to let someone else know us.

Another way we avoid the intimacy we fear is by focusing on the need of a sexual high. Whether in a long-term relationship or not, our thinking that sex is love limits our chance for true intimacy and connection with another person. Healthy sex is an expression of an intimacy that already exists; when we use it as a tool to become intimate, we are almost always disappointed in the results.

Action to Take

Set aside relationship dramas that distract you from having to face your own emptiness. Can you practice staying connected and enjoying the meaningful pleasures of true intimacy?

The Practice of Being Nonreactive

Were you reactive today? Did you spend time, thought, and energy on how you've been wronged? Do you have tension, disease, or judgment about how someone else treated you?

We can most likely make a great argument to justify our reactions, but those who throw away their resources in this way have little left over for growth and spiritual awakening. Perhaps we are right and they are wrong, but still, no matter how justified we may be, we are wasting energy. When we take things personally and/or are oversensitive, we become self-righteous, and this is a huge diversion from our path of personal development. It creates anxiety in us, and our strength is undermined.

Our self-importance requires that we spend most of our lives offended by someone. How much better would it be to let go of the sensitivity, our puffed-up righteousness, and our superiority and simply practice serenity in a moment of difficulty? How much more graceful would it be not to judge the imperfections in others and in ourselves? When we do this, we are better people. Our personal force and energy can be funneled into a life worth living.

Action to Take

Know that reactivity is a choice, not a reflex we are powerless against.

The Practice of Being Honest with Yourself

There is a saying, "Every time I close the door on reality, it comes in through the back window." Many of us close the door on the reality of who we really are and the life we really live. We explain away our lives and our behaviors, hiding the truth with our sugar-coated behavior and language. Yet reality eventually comes through the back window in the form of anxiety, drama, and chaos. Over the years I've seen so many people who pride themselves on their self-honesty but are unable to see the inconsistency that is flowing in through the back window of their lives.

Truthfulness is a pillar of spiritual awakening. We cannot grow without it. We do not define or create the truth—we accept it and surrender to it. The truth is sometimes painful, but it is the pain of rebirth of a real man or a real woman.

Action to Take

Resolve today to be fully honest with yourself about your motivations, your behaviors, and your responsibility in the dramas of your life, and be clear about the effects.

The Practice of Equanimity

The *Bhagavad-Gita* states that "a restless man's mind is so strongly shaken in the grip of the senses . . . truly I think the wind is no wilder." As quick as flicking a switch, our passions can cause us to abandon our reasoning powers. We can so easily let go of our conscience, values, and better judgment in order to pursue our lusts.

We all know about the ferocious hurricanelike winds of obsessive, compulsive, and addictive reactions and behaviors. But now we are on a path, and we are learning that equanimity comes from melding our sensual nature with our mind and our morals. As we become more centered, we can feel the wild winds of our senses with-

out getting swept away by them. We have our intuition, our mind, and the guiding spirit within to bring us back when we get sucked into the thunderous storms of turbulent times.

Action to Take

When the winds of emotional need or desire blow through, use it as an opportunity to practice equanimity. Secure yourself to a steady and calm center, and you'll notice how much easier it is to simply let the storm ride on by.

The Practice of Not Resisting Change

Many of us have a selfish mind-set around change. When the path gets rocky or unfamiliar, we say, "Grab the bull by the horns!" or "Fix this!" We do this because we don't understand what change really is, and we resist it. When we launch into control mode and try to change ourselves by our own methods—setting goals, "lifting ourselves up by the bootstraps"—we end up recycling and reawakening our problems.

At a certain point, we learn that unconditional surrender is a far superior approach to life than our compulsion to control. The rewards of getting healthy are ours, if we yield to living by the principles that set us free and provide ongoing transformation. However, we must also know that transformation does not come on our timetable. It happens in God's time. We do our part when we surrender and allow change to remold us. It's important that we earnestly give our hearts over to accepting change and growing from it, rather than resisting it or trying to control it. Positive change comes not when we declare, "I've earned this," but when we are ready and willing to receive it.

Action to Take

Ask yourself: What change are you resisting? In what transition or circumstance in your life are you trying to control the outcome? What would happen if you stopped trying to control it and just flowed with it?

The Practice of Relationship

Actions create effects, most notably in the realm of relationships. Our behavior, actions, and attitudes have a way of boomeranging back to us, and we tend to get what we do. If what we do is launch into anger, shake our fists, and scream a lot, what we get is a list of people who don't want to be around us. If what we do is withdraw and put up walls to keep others out, what we get is a deep sense of loneliness and a feeling of being defective or unlovable. If what we do is get involved with people who cannot hold up their end of a healthy relationship based on a higher

love, what we get is a broken heart. These scenarios can repeat themselves again and again and again.

On the other side of things, if we give energy to making ourselves healthier, more whole, and less selfish people, we become genuinely ready for relationships that can work for us. If we consistently work our inner revolution, what we get is an inspired and healthy life, filled with other inspired and healthy people.

We all need to mature to the point where, rather than complaining about the effects, we spend time looking at our attitudes and behaviors that have caused them. Then we can see that we really do have options for what we can manifest in our relationships and our lives.

Action to Take

The next time your instinct is to blame someone else for a fracture or drama in your relationship, notice your own contribution to the problem, and what attitudes or behaviors you might have generated in order to cause it.

The Practice of Slowing Down

What do we really want? What are we looking for? Often we feel restless, driven, and even compulsive in our doing, but to what end? What are we really seeking in all our frantic grasping and doing? Becoming conscious, slowing down, and slamming on the brakes just enough during the day gives us a much better chance of knowing what we are looking for, and of ultimately finding it.

Each day, we can slow down by taking time for meditation, prayer, solitude, and silence in order to connect with what is really in our heart. Sometimes it may be that we need to call a friend to make a connection and create the conscious contact in order to reanchor. Perhaps we read something meaningful to give us soulful ideas to contemplate and assimilate. We could take a walk or get into nature to give ourselves some space from the things that absorb us. We give so much power to the events in our lives that we often miss out on the transformation and wisdom that comes from the space between events.

Action to Take

Remember that if you are looking for something and you're traveling too fast, you'll pass it by.

The Practice of Forgiveness

Many of us are carrying around unfinished resentments about the things in our past. Perhaps things in our lives should have been better; the fact is, they weren't. We walk around with these resentments like a low-grade toothache, and they grind away

at our hearts and keep us in our heads. We get stuck in mental chatter, preoccupation, and fantasy, reliving conversations and situations in our heads. Essentially, the word *re-sentment* means to re-send something again and again. Our anger is a sign that we keep playing the same old tapes over and over in our heads.

The truth may be that in the past we got what others gave us, but now we get what we give to ourselves. Usually, we create what we focus on, and if we continue to focus on where we were wronged, we keep ourselves stuck. It's hard to be spiritual and full of anger at the same time. Since we do eventually get what we focus on, we may as well aim for forgiveness.

The spiritual path promises many rewards, but it does not promise to be easy. We must search our conscience for resentments and face them. No one can really grow while holding on to resentments, old angers, and hatred. When we hold these things in our hearts, we block the dark corners of our souls from receiving the light of renewal that we need. As we forgive through the willingness of our mind, we no longer need to reserve those secret pockets within ourselves for the energy of power and resentment.

Nothing can be held back! We must be willing to wave the white flag of our ego and surrender it all—even if we do not know how. We cannot stop being resentful by simply deciding to stop; there is no instant cure here. Forgiveness can happen only when we are willing to be honest with ourselves and completely humble.

Action to Take

Ask yourself: What resentment am I carrying around? At whom is it aimed? What people, events, and issues am I resentful of in my life? Am I willing to 'fess up, forgive, and clean the slate—even if I don't know how?

The Practice of Coming Clean

There is a saying that we are as sick as the secrets we keep. Keeping secrets from others can make us lonely and can even make us physically ill. Secrets are like poison in our system: They build up as toxic shame and will release in some sort of sideways behavior. We may turn to food, alcohol, drugs, sex, or emotional drama, but somehow we will act it out because that energy has to go somewhere. Secrets are links in our chains of slavery to self-betraying patterns of behavior, including addictions, codependency, and compulsive behavior.

As we become healthy, we strive to live a life of honesty as it relates to not just ourselves but to others as well. When we come clean with the people in our lives, we realize it's as though we were holding our breath for a long time and we are finally able to exhale. Suddenly there is a great sense of relief and freedom.

Yet honesty may not mean telling everything to everyone. Therefore, we need to develop the spiritual maturity to choose what, when, and in whom to confide. We need to develop internal limits around when to express something and when not to, and to remember that honesty without compassion is not really honesty, but hostility.

Action to Take

Get clear about any secrets you've been keeping. Commit to being true to your intuition about what you need to discuss with others in your life, and when to hold back. Your right intention will guide you.

Yoga Practices

Integration

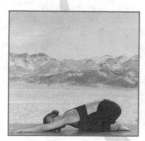
Child's Pose

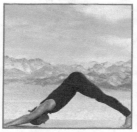
Downward Facing Dog
(Adho Mukha Svanasana)

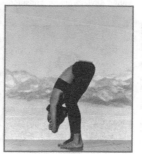
Ragdoll

Sun Salutation/Vinyasa A

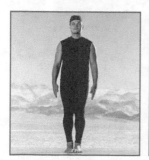
Samasthiti

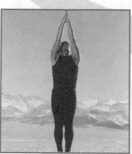
Mountain Pose (Tadasana)

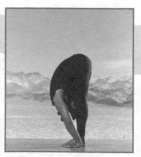
Standing Forward Bend
(Uttanasana)

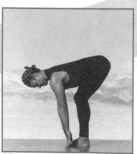
Halfway Lift
(Urdhva Mukha Uttanasana)

Sun Salutation/Vinyasa A (continued)

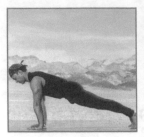

High Push-Up (Dandasana)

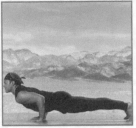

Low Push-Up
(Chaturanga Dandasana)

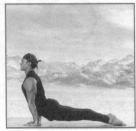

Upward Facing Dog
(Urdhva Mukha Svanasana)

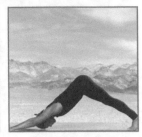

Downward Facing Dog
(Adho Mukha Svanasana)

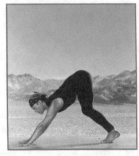

Jump Forward, starting position

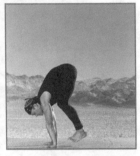

Jump Forward, finishing position

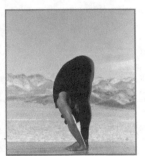

Halfway Lift
(Urdhva Mukha Uttanasana)

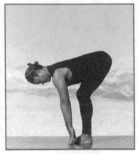

Standing Forward Bend
(Uttanasana)

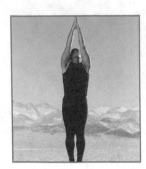

Mountain Pose (Tadasana)

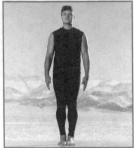

Samathiti

YOGA PRACTICES

Sun Salutation/Vinyasa B

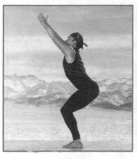

Thunderbolt (Utkatasana)

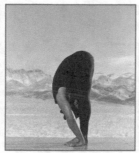

Standing Forward Bend (Uttanasana)

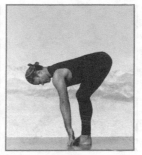

Halfway Lift (Urdhva Mukha Uttanasana)

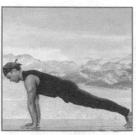

High Push-Up (Dandasana)

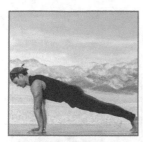

Low Push-Up (Chaturanga Dandasana)

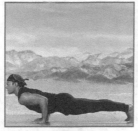

Upward Facing Dog (Urdhva Mukha Svanasana)

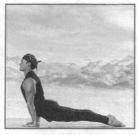

Downward Facing Dog (Adho Mukha Svanasana)

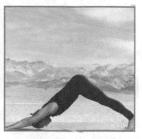

Warrior I (Virabhadrasana I), right foot forward

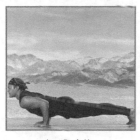

High Push-Up (Dandasana)

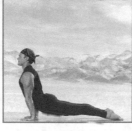

Low Push-Up (Chaturanga Dandasana)

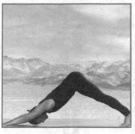

Upward Facing Dog (Urdhva Mukha Svanasana)

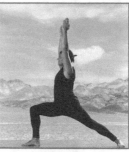

Downward Facing Dog (Adho Mukha Svanasana)

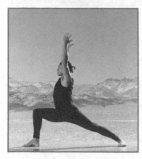

Warrior I (Virabhadrasana I), left foot forward

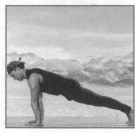

High Push-Up (Dandasana)

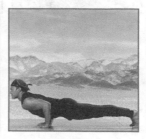

Low Push-Up (Chaturanga Dandasana)

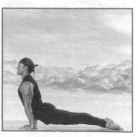

Upward Facing Dog (Urdhva Mukha Svanasana)

Sun Salutation/Vinyasa B (continued)

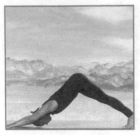

Downward Facing Dog
(Adho Mukha Svanasana)

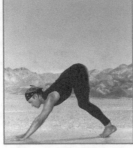

Jump Forward, starting position

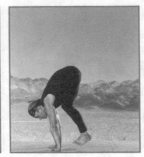

Jump Forward, finishing position

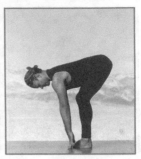

Halfway Lift
(Urdhva Mukha Uttanasana)

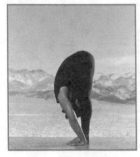

Standing Forward Bend
(Uttanasana)

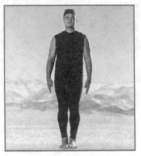

Samasthiti

Closing Sequence

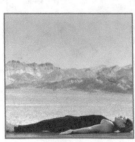

Savasana

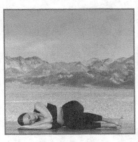

Closing sequence I

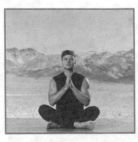

Closing sequence II

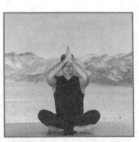

Closing sequence III

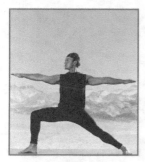

Warrior II (Virabhadrasana II)

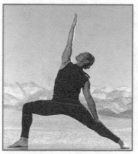

Reverse Warrior
(Parivrtta Virabhadrasana II)

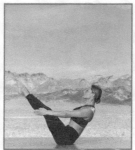

Boat Pose (Navasana)

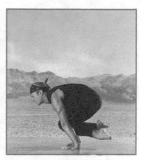

Boat Pose (Navasana), step 2

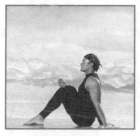

Seated Half-Pigeon
(Urdhva Mukha Sukhasana)

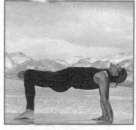

Three-Legged Tabletop
(Arda Purvottanasana)

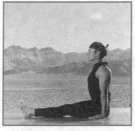

The Staff (Dandasana)

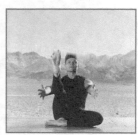

Single-Legged Boat
(Ekapadanavasana)

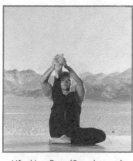

Lifted Leg Pose (Crunchasana)

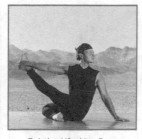

Twisting Lifted Leg Pose
(Parivrtta Crunchasana)

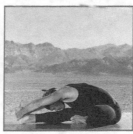

Easy Forward Bend
(Janu Sirsasana)

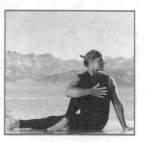

Straight Leg Seated Twist
(Parivrtta Marichyasana)

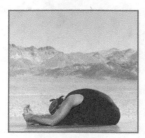

Seated Forward Bend
(Paschimotonasana)

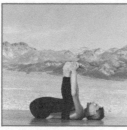

Dead Bug Pose (Urdhva Mukha
Upavista Konasana)

From Week 2

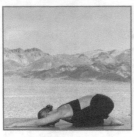

Child's Pose

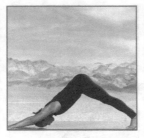

Downward Facing Dog
(Adho Mukha Svanasana)

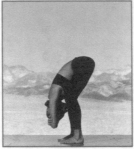

Ragdoll

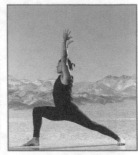

Warrior I (Virabhadrasana I),
left foot forward

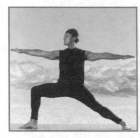

Warrior II (Virabhadrasana II)

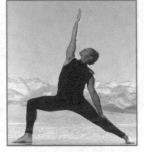

Reverse Warrior
(Parivrtta Virabhadrasana II)

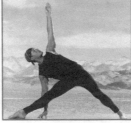

Triangle (Trikonasana)

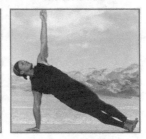

Side Plank (Vasisthasana)

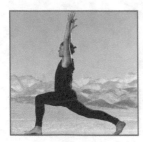

Crescent Lunge (Anjaneyasana)

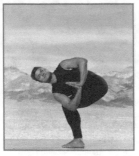

Prayer Twist (Parivrtta), step 1

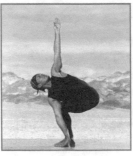

Prayer Twist (Parivrtta), step 2

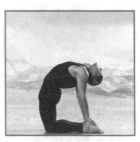

Camel (Ustrasana)

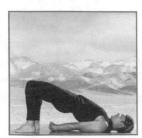

Bridge (Setubandasana)

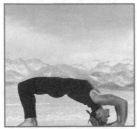

Wheel (Urdhva Dhanurasana),
step 1, preparation

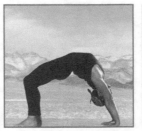

Wheel (Urdhva Dhanurasana),
step 2

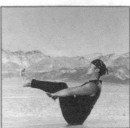

Easy Boat Pose (Sukhanavasana)

YOGA PRACTICES

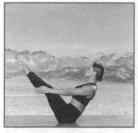

Boat Pose (Navasana)

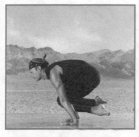

Boat Pose (Navasana), step 2

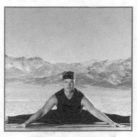

Sitting Splits Pose
(Urdhvakonasana)

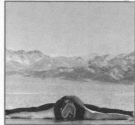

Bowing Splits Pose
(Upavistakonasana)

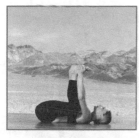

Dead Bug Pose (Urdhva Mukha
Upavista Konasana)

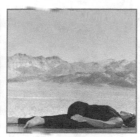

Supine Twist

From Week 3

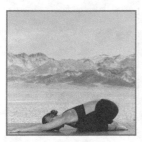

Child's Pose

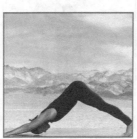

Downward Facing Dog
(Adho Mukha Svanasana)

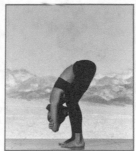

Ragdoll

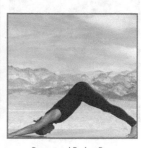

Downward Facing Dog
(Adho Mukha Svanasana)

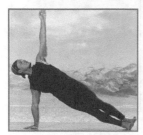

Side Plank (Vasisthasana)

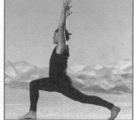

Crescent Lunge (Anjaneyasana)

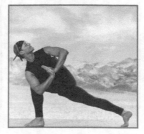

Revolving Crescent Lunge
(Parivrtta Alanasana) step 1

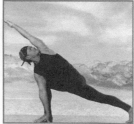

Revolving Crescent Lunge
(Parivrtta Alanasana) step 2

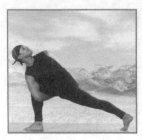

Revolving Crescent Lunge
(Parivrtta Alanasana) step 3

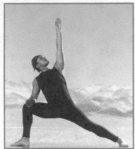

Extended Side Angle
(Utthita Parsvakonasana)

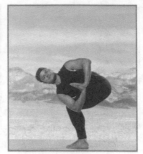

Prayer Twist (Parivrtta), step 1

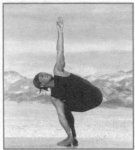

Prayer Twist (Parivrtta), step 2

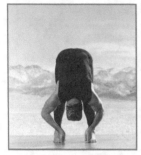

Gorilla Pose (Padhastasana)

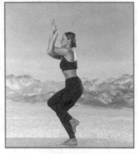

Eagle (Garudasana)

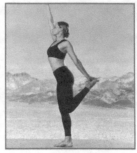

Dancer's Pose (Natarajasana),
step 1, preparation

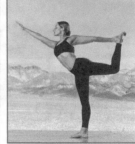

Dancer's Pose
(Natarajasana), step 2

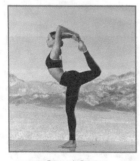

Dancer's Pose
(Natarajasana), step 3

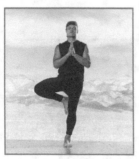

Tree Pose (Vrksasana), step 1

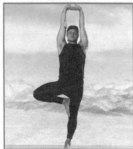

Tree Pose (Vrksasana), step 2

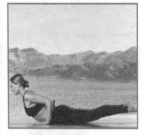

Locust (Salabhasana)

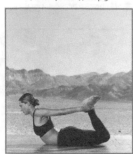

Bow Pose (Dhanurasana)

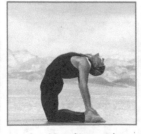

Camel Pose (Ustrasana)

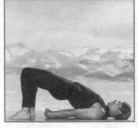

Bridge Pose (Setubandasana)

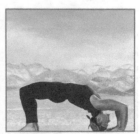

Wheel (Urdhva Dhanurasana),
step 1, preparation

YOGA PRACTICES

238

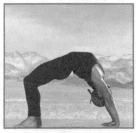

Wheel (Urdhva Dhanurasana),
step 2

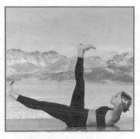

Scissor Legs

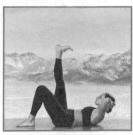

Scissor Legs Modification

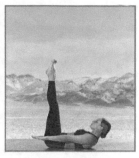

60/30 Lift (1)

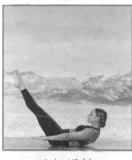

60/30 Lift (2)

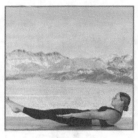

60/30 Lift (3)

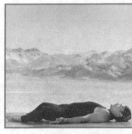

Supta Baddha Konasana

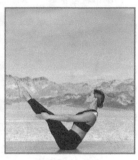

Boat Pose (Navasana)

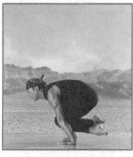

Boat Pose (Navasana), step 2

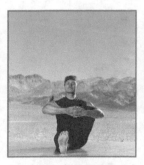

Rock the Baby (Vinyaspadmasana)

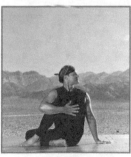

Bent Leg Seated Twist
(Marichyasana)

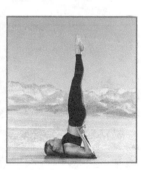

Shoulder Stand (Sarvangasana)

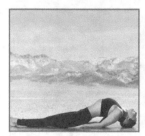

Fish Pose (Matsyasana)

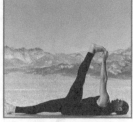

Supine Leg Raise, Front
(Supta Ardhva Padangushasana)

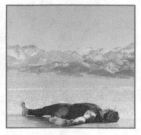

Supine Leg Raise, Side

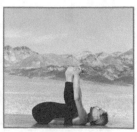

Dead Bug (Urdhva Mukha
Upavista Konasana)

From Week 3 (continued)

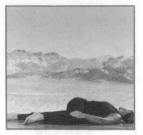

Supine Twist

From Week 4

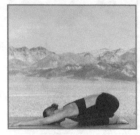

Child's Pose

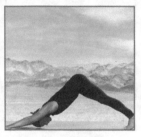

Downward Facing Dog
(Adho Mukha Svanasana)

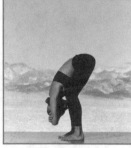

Ragdoll

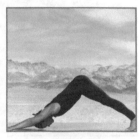

Downward Facing Dog
(Adho Mukha Svanasana)

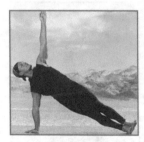

Side Plank (Vasisthasana)

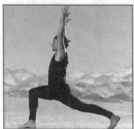

Crescent Lunge (Anjaneyasana)

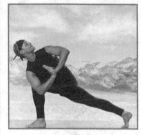

Parivrtta Alanasana, step 1

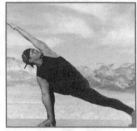

Revolving Crescent Lunge
(Parivrta Alanasana), step 2

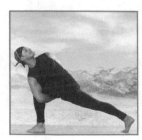

Parivrtta Alanasana, step 3

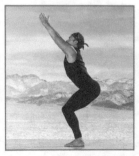

Thunderbolt (Utkatasana)

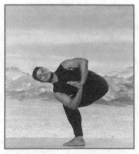

Prayer Twist (Parivrtta), step 1

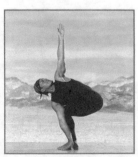

Prayer Twist (Parivrtta), step 2

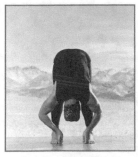

Gorilla Pose (Padhastasana)

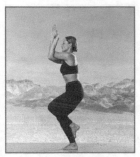

Eagle Pose (Garudasana)

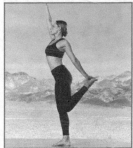

Dancer's Pose (Natarajasana), step 1, preparation

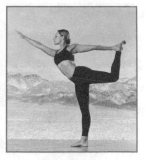

Dancer's Pose (Natarajasana), step 2

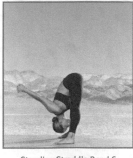

Dancer's Pose (Natarajasana), step 3

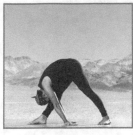

Tree Pose (Vrksasana), step 1

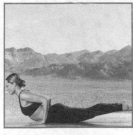

Tree Pose (Vrksasana), step 2

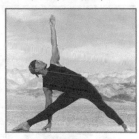

Triangle (Trikonasana)

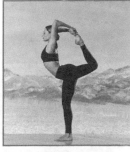

Standing Straddle Bend C (Prasarita C)

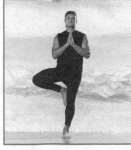

Pyramid (Parsvottanasana)

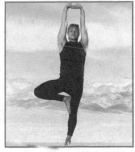

Locust Pose (Salabhasana)

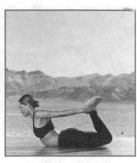

Bow Pose (Dhanurasana)

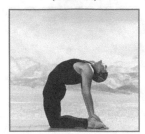

Camel Pose (Ustrasana)

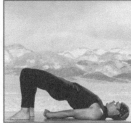

Bridge Pose (Setubandasana)

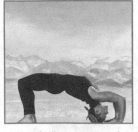

Wheel (Urdhva Dhanurasana), step 1, preparation

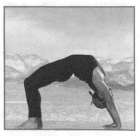

Wheel (Urdhva Dhanurasana), step 2

From Week 4 (continued)

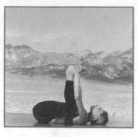

Dead bug (Urdhva Mukha
Upavista Konasana)

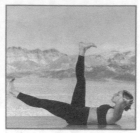

Scissor Legs (1)

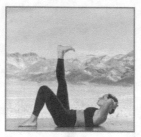

Scissor Legs (2)

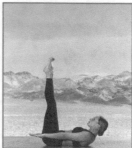

60/30 Lift (1)

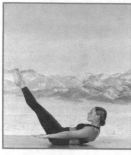

60/30 Lift (2)

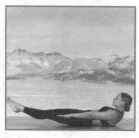

60/30 Lift (3)

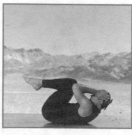

Abdominal Twists (step 1)

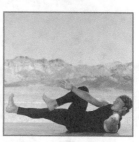

Abdominal Twist (step 2)

YOGA PRACTICES

242

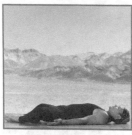

Supta Baddha Konasana

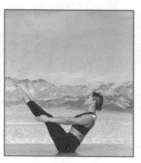

Boat Pose (Navasana)

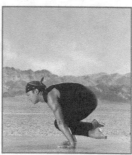

Boat Pose (Navasana), step 2

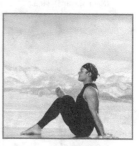

Seated Half Pigeon
(Urdhva Mukha Sukhasana)

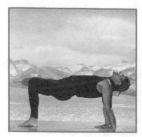

Three-Legged Tabletop
(Arda Purvottanasana)

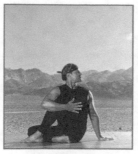

Bent Leg Seated Twist
(Marichyasana)

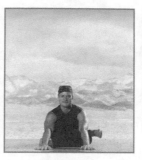

Double Pigeon
(Dwapada Rajakapotoasana)

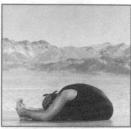

Seated Forward Bend
(Paschimotonasana)

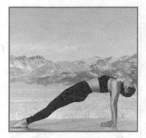

Tabletop (Purvottanasana)

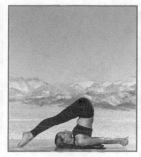

Shoulder Stand (Sarvangasana)

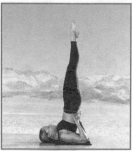

Plow (Halasana)

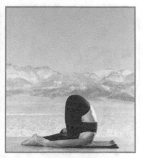

Deaf Man's Pose (Karnapidasana)

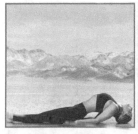

Fish Pose (Matsyasana)

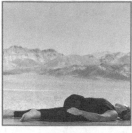

Supine Twist

From Week 5

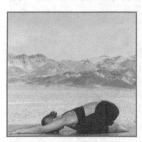

Child's Pose

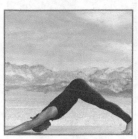

Downward Facing Dog
(Adho Mukha Svanasana)

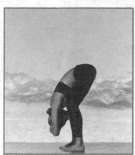

Ragdoll

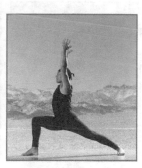

Warrior I (Virabhadrasana I),
left foot forward

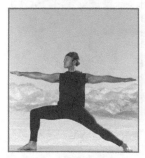

Warrior II (Virabhadrasana II)

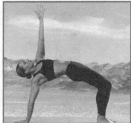

Flipped Downward Dog

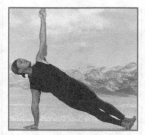

Side Plank (Vasisthasana)

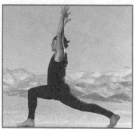

Crescent Lunge (Anjaneyasana)

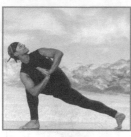

Revolving Crescent Lunge
(Parivrtta Alanasana), step 1

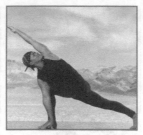

Revolving Crescent Lunge
(Parivrtta Alanasana), step 2

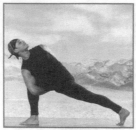

Revolving Crescent Lunge
(Parivrtta Alanasana), step 3

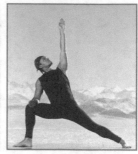

Extended Side Angle
(Utthita Parsvakonasana)

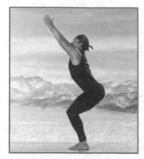

Thunderbolt (Utkatasana)

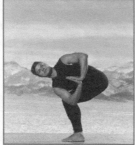

Prayer Twist (Parivrtta), step 1

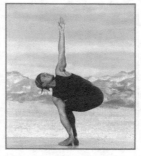

Prayer Twist (Parivrtta), step 2

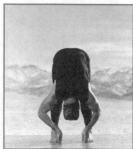

Gorilla Pose (Padhastasana)

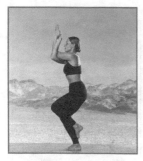

Eagle Pose (Garudasana)

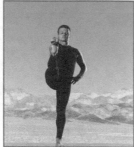

Standing Leg Raise, Front (Utthita
Hasta Padangusthasana A)

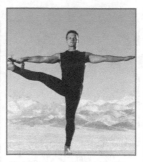

Standing Leg Raise, Side (Utthita
Hasta Padangusthasana B)

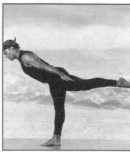

Airplane (Dekasana)

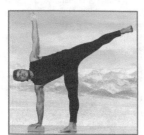

Half Moon (Ardhachandrasana)

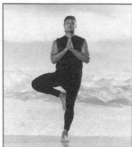

Tree Pose (Vrksasana), step 1

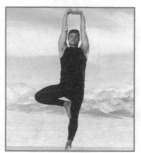

(Vrksasana), step 2

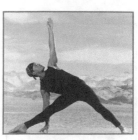

Triangle (Trikonasana)

YOGA PRACTICES

244

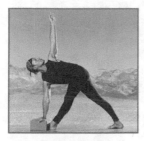

Twisting Triangle
(Parivrtta Trikonasana)

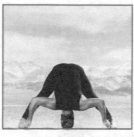

Standing Straddle Bend D
(Prasarita D)

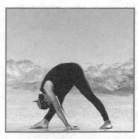

Pyramid Pose (Parsvottanasana)

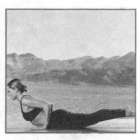

Locust Pose (Salabhasana)

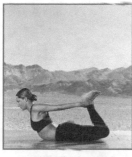

Bow Pose (Dhanurasana)

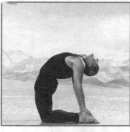

Camel Pose (Ustrasana)

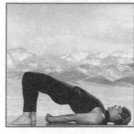

Bridge Pose (Setubandasana)

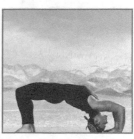

Wheel (Urdhva Dhanurasana),
step 1, preparation

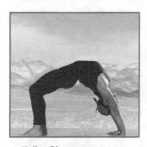

Urdhva Dhanurasana, step 2

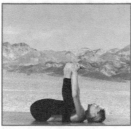

Dead Bug (Urdhva Mukha
Upavista Konasana)

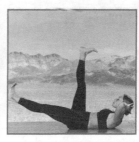

Scissor Legs Modification

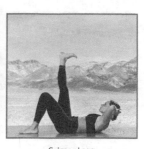

Scissor Legs

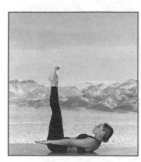

60/30 Lift (1)

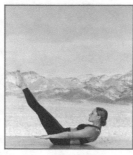

60/30 Lift (2)

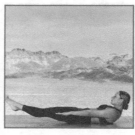

60/30 Lift (3)

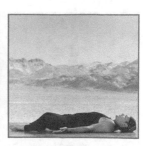

Supta Baddha Konasana

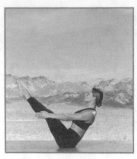

Boat Pose (Navasana)

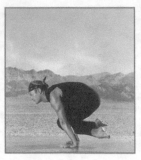

Boat Pose (Navasana), step 2

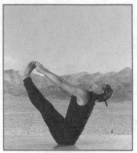

Upward Facing Boat Pose
(Urdhva Padangushasana)

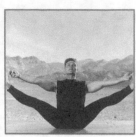

Wide Balancing Boat Pose
(Merudandasana)

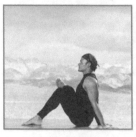

Seated Half Pigeon
(Urdhva Mukha Sukhasana)

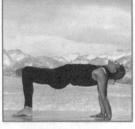

Three-Legged Tabletop
(Arda Purvottanasana)

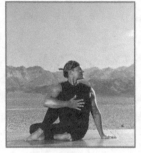

Bent Leg Seated Twist
(Marichyasana)

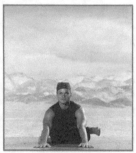

Double Pigeon
(Dwapada Rajakapotoasana)

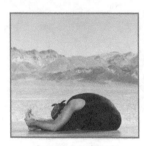

Seated Forward Bend
(Paschimotonasana)

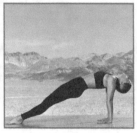

Tabletop (Purvottanasana)

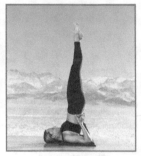

Shoulder Stand (Sarvangasana)

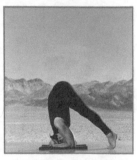

Headstand (Sirsasana), step 1

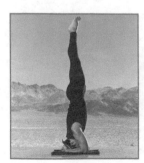

Headstand (Sirsasana), step 2

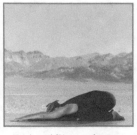

Headstand (Sirsasana), step 3

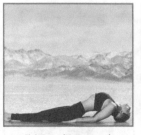

Fish Pose (Matsyasana)

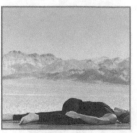

Supine Twist

YOGA PRACTICES

246

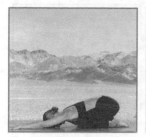

Child's Pose

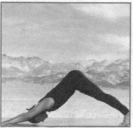

Downward Facing Dog
(Adho Mukha Svanasana)

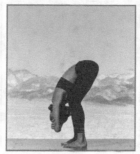

Ragdoll

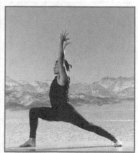

Warrior I (Virabhadrasana I),
left foot forward

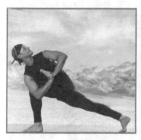

Warrior II (Virabhadrasana II)

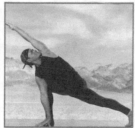

Flipped Downward Dog
(Urdhva Mukha Svanasana)

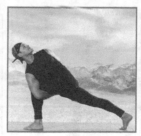

Side Plank (Vasisthasana)

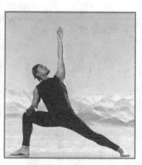

Crescent Lunge (Anjaneyasana)

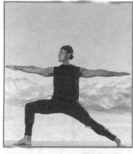

Revolving Crescent Lunge
(Parivrtta Alanasana), step 1

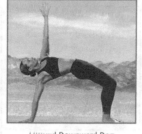

Revolving Crescent Lunge
(Parivrtta Alanasana), step 2

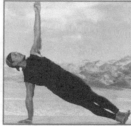

Revolving Crescent Lunge
(Parivrtta Alanasana), step 3

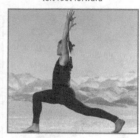

Extended Side Angle
(Utthita Parsvakonasana)

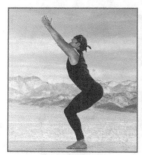

Thunderbolt (Utkatasana)

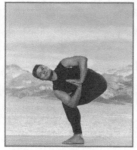

Prayer Twist (Parivrtta), step 1

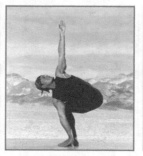

Prayer Twist (Parivrtta), step 2

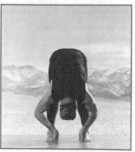

Gorilla Pose (Padhastasana)

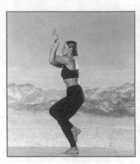

Eagle Pose (Garudasana)

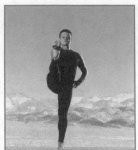

Standing Leg Raise, Front (Utthita Hasta Padangusthasana A)

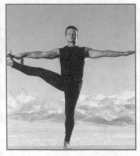

Standing Leg Raise, Side Standing Leg Raise, Side (Utthita Hasta Padangusthasana B)

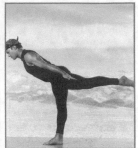

Airplane (Dekasana)

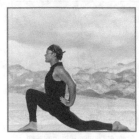

Deep Hip Lunge (Ardha Virabhadrasana), step 1

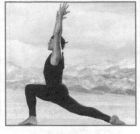

Deep Hip Lunge (Ardha Virabhadrasana), step 2

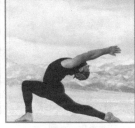

Deep Hip Lunge (Ardha Virabhadrasana), step 3

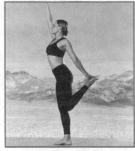

Dancer's Pose (Natarajasana), step 1, preparation

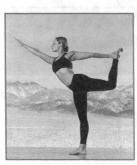

Dancer's Pose (Natarajasana), step 2

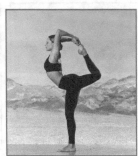

Dancer's Pose (Natarajasana), step 3

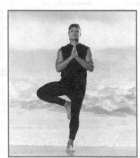

Tree Pose (Vrksasana), step 1

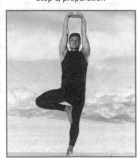

Tree Pose (Vrksasana), step 2

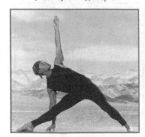

Triangle (Trikonasana)

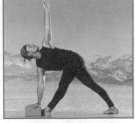

Twisting Triangle (Parivrtta Trikonasana)

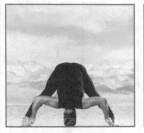

Standing Straddle Bend D (Prasarita D)

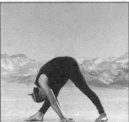

Pyramid Pose (Parsvottanasana)

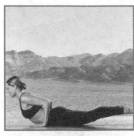

Locust Pose (Salabhasana)

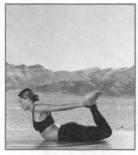

Bow Pose (Dhanurasana)

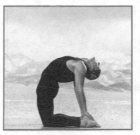

Camel Pose (Ustrasana)

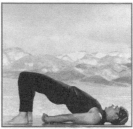

Bridge Pose (Setubandasana)

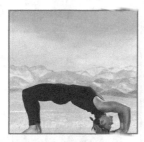

Wheel (Urdhva Dhanurasana),
step 1, preparation

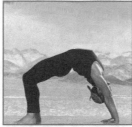

Wheel (Urdhva Dhanurasana),
step 2

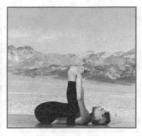

Dead Bug (Urdhva Mukha
Upavista Konasana)

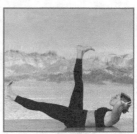

Scissor Legs

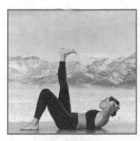

Scissor Legs Modification

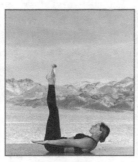

60/30 Lift (1)

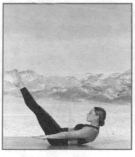

60/30 Lift (2)

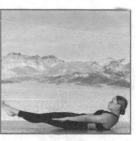

60/30 Lift (3)

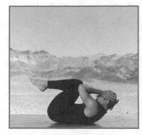

Abdominal Twist (step 1)

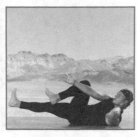

Abdominal Twist (step 2)

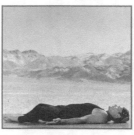

Supta Baddha Konasana

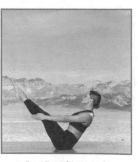

Boat Pose (Navasana)

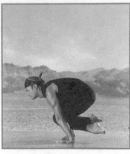

Boat Pose (Navasana), step 2

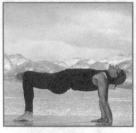

Seated Half Pigeon
(Urdhva Mukha Sukhasana)

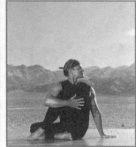

Three-legged Tabletop
(Arda Purvottanasana)

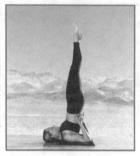

Bent Leg Seated Twist
(Marichyasana)

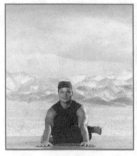

Double Pigeon
(Dwapada Rajakapotoasana)

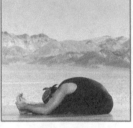

Seated Forward Bend
(Paschimotonasana)

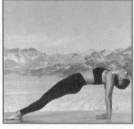

Tabletop (Purvottanasana)

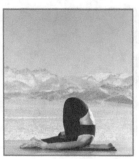

Shoulder Stand (Sarvangasana)

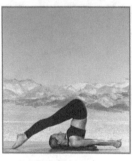

Plow (Halasana)

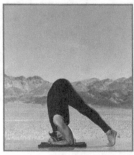

Deaf Man's Pose (Karnapidasana)

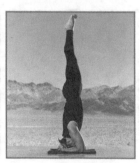

Headstand (Sirsasana), step 1

Headstand (Sirsasana), step 2

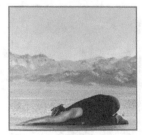

Headstand (Sirsasana), step 3

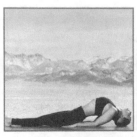

Fish Pose (Matsyasana)

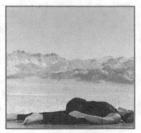

Supine Twist

YOGA PRACTICES

CONGRATULATIONS!
You've Taken the First Step.

Now, Continue Your Personal Revolution and Open the Door to Infinite Possibilities.

Baptiste Power Yoga Institute's mission is to empower you to live your life with a renewed personal force. We design our products, programs, and classes so that they will strengthen your journey and transform your life in a way that is accessible, sensible, and fun. Take this powerful process to the next level by purchasing a product, or if you want to take a deep plunge into radical, invigorating change, you could attend one of our weekend or weeklong programs.

Videos, DVDs, Audio CDs Unlike Any You've Ever Experienced:

We've created our video and audio products as a way for you to bring the transformational process to life. Our products are a wonderful way for you to take the principles and practices you read about in this book to the next level. We offer various videos, DVDs, CDs, and products for the beginning to the experienced student. Please visit www.baronbaptiste.com or call 1-800-936-9642 for our latest selection of products and offerings.

Personal Revolution Teacher Training Programs:

We offer various Intensive Teacher Training programs, for those who are aspiring to teach Baptiste Power Vinyasa Yoga. At Baron Baptiste's Teacher Trainings, whether an introductory or advanced training, you will learn the foundational principles and practices of teaching Baptiste Power Vinyasa Yoga, through an approach that focuses on personal transformation on all levels. During these trainings, you grow as a teacher and discover the extraordinary within yourself. Potent personal and professional growth is realized. This process awakens you to deeper insights and new perceptions. It will teach you how to apply newly discovered truths to your life—both in and out of the classroom. Call us at 1-800-936-9642 or visit www.baronbaptiste.com to see which training is right for you. Trainings offered in the United States and worldwide.

Personal Revolution Weekends and Bootcamps:

Attending a Baptiste Personal Revolution Weekend or Bootcamp is an opportunity to transform your life forever. These empowering programs awaken the sacred within your body and soul. Baron Baptiste offers you the ultimate life transformation program. You will emerge lighter, focused, and empowered. Learn how to excavate your ideal practice, free your true self, and transform your life. Celebrate your personal revolution! Call us at 1-800-936-9642 or visit www. baronbaptiste.com for our latest schedule of events.

Baptiste Power Yoga Institutes:

The Baptiste Power Vinyasa Yoga Studios are built on a simple principle that everyone can do power yoga, regardless of age, strength, or weight. Our classes will lead you to build and maintain a physical and spiritual vitality which will completely change your life.

Each Baptiste studio offers our classic All-Levels and Power Yoga Basic classes for students of all different levels of experience and fitness abilities. All of our classes have a powerful physical component coupled with an intellectual understanding in which to continue your personal revolution! Visit www.baronbaptiste.com for studio locations.

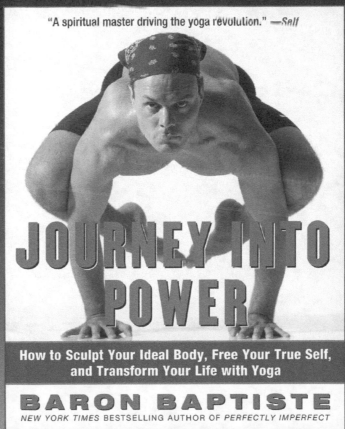
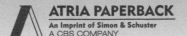